KAMA
SUTRA

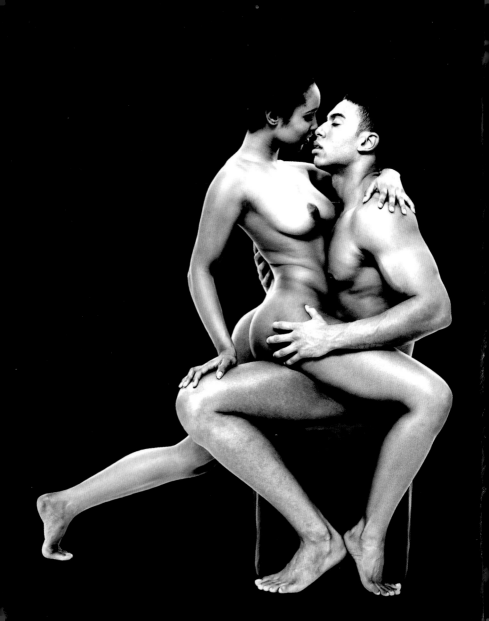

KAMA SUTRA

SUTRA

A POSITION A DAY
365 *DAYS A YEAR*

LONDON, NEW YORK, MELBOURNE, MUNICH, AND DELHI

Author Claudia Blake
Managing Editor Dawn Henderson
Managing Art Editor Christine Keilty
Publisher Peggy Vance
Art Director Peter Luff
Preproducer Andy Hilliard
Producer Oliver Jeffreys
Creative Technical Support Tom Morse

First American Edition, 2014

Published in the United States by
DK Publishing, 345 Hudson Street, New York, New York 10014

17 18   10 9 8 7 6

019—192988—Jan/14

Published in Great Britain by Dorling Kindersley Limited.

A catalog record for this book is available from the Library of Congress.

ISBN 978-1-4654-1582-0

DK books are available at special discounts when purchased in bulk for sales promotions, premiums,
fund-raising, or educational use. For details, contact: DK Publishing Special Markets, 345 Hudson
Street, New York, New York 10014 or SpecialSales@dk.com.

Color reproduction by Altaimage
Printed and bound in China

Discover more at www.dk.com

Contents

Introduction

Since time out of mind, we've loved spicing up our sex lives with a little variety. Have you ever wanted to dazzle a new lover with your wicked invention? Or to refresh the long-cherished intimacy you hold with the familiar love of your life? Or to try something totally new just for the fun of it? As it turns out, so did our ancestors.

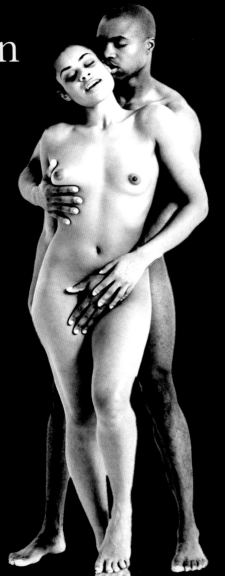

INTRODUCTION

Here, you'll find a position for every day of the
year, inspired not only by the most famous love text
in history but by other classic authors. Who hasn't
heard of the Kama Sutra? Written sometime
between the second and fifth centuries by the great
yogi Mallanaga Vatsyayana, its aim was not just to
share naughty secrets but also to reflect on the
whole nature of pleasure, love, and how to live a
fulfilling life. A grand work indeed, but not the only
word on the subject: In these pages, you'll also find
tips from other classics—the Smaradipika, the
Ananga Ranga, the Panchasayaka, the
Ratikallonlini—books written by poets, scholars
and philosophers to enlighten lovers across the
ages. If all that sounds scholarly, don't worry:
Yourself and your partner are all you need to bring
to the table... or bed, floor, staircase,
or anywhere else you choose.

INTRODUCTION

People are sexy creatures, whenever or wherever
they're born, and we love to experiment. We all
know that different positions are one way to shake
things up: Sex is a physical conversation and the
stance you strike at the beginning can do a lot for
your tone. But there's more to it than just different
twists and angles. Human beings are creative, and
we like to work together making new and beautiful
things. As the ancient writers taught us, sex can be
part of that: To try new ideas in bed is to sculpt
with sensation, to paint with love. Artists of former
times knew that sex could be an art.

INTRODUCTION

There are many ways you can read this book. You can leaf through, looking for a new favorite and trying whatever catches your eye. You can take on the huge and hilarious challenge of attempting one position every day—and whether you succeed or not, there's no question you and your partner will be happier, funnier, and closer for giving it a shot. If you're after something specific, you can also flip to the end, where you'll find a Random Selector pointing you toward our particular recommendations for whatever mood you're in.

Some of these positions are sensual, sleepy, or spiritual caresses. Some of them are limb-bending, brow-raising feats to make you feel tingly all over. All of them are a door to a creative playground where you and your lover can run wild.

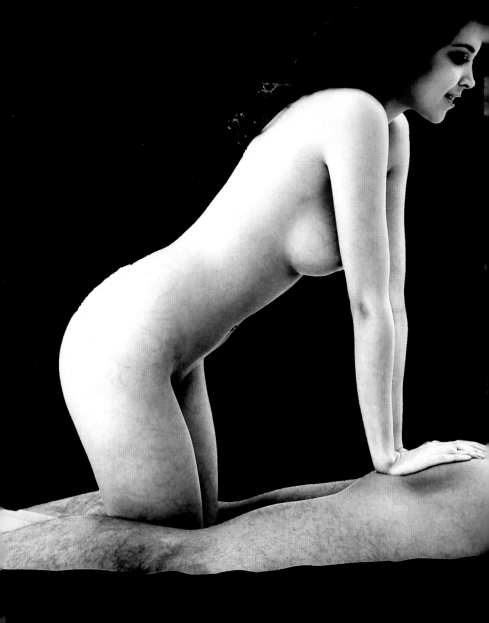

The Positions

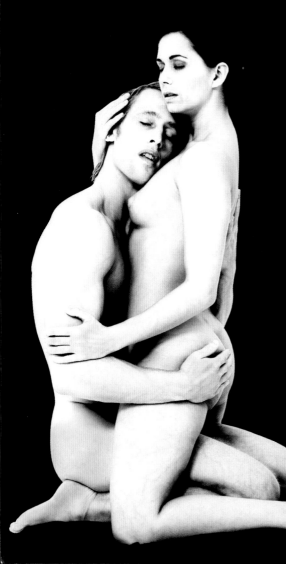

Meditate to the beat of your goddess's heart

a loving and sensual full-body caress

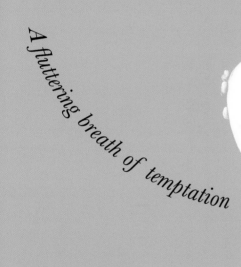

A fluttering breath of temptation

the Kama Sutra says this is for young virgins, but don't let that stop you

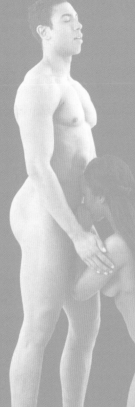

The delicious
full-mouthed swallow

a timeless way
to a man's heart

*Treasure her clitoris with
delicate skill*

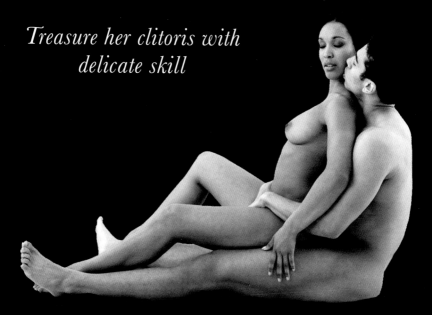

lightly massage with
fingertips on either side,
moving in gentle counterpoint

Bring all your pride to this graceful seat

the wide-set posture
makes the woman's back
rise straight and haughty

*Twine together in
                unthinking bliss*

eyes closed and heads
averted, experience
pure sensation

DAY 7 THE KNIGHT'S SALUTE

Courtly virility no woman can resist

no need to kiss chastely—
let your lips and tongue
plead your case

DAY 8 KSHOBAKA (STIRRING)

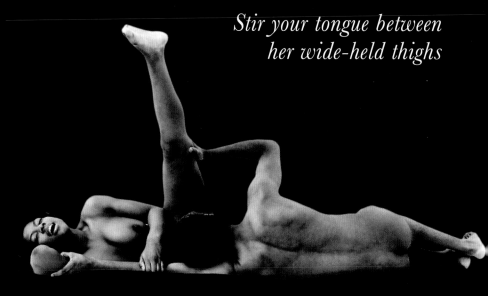

Stir your tongue between her wide-held thighs

the Kama Sutra describes this lapping movement as drinking at her sacred fountain

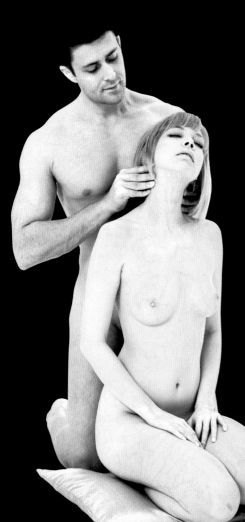

Succumb to a state
of pure nurture

fingertips at the
base of the skull
are chaste, but
astonishingly intimate

So happy together you could dance on air

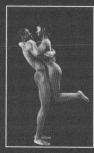

a wonderful way to reunite,
no matter how long you've
been parted

He sees, he yearns …
he waits for her word

displaying
her pretty yoni
and flexible body
at the same time,
this is one for the
true show-off

*Twine thigh-to-genital and
twist in mutual delight*

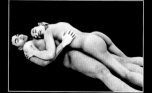

a sleepy, sensuous caress for
lovers newly acquainted

Raise a salute to your passion

she grows
light-headed
with sensation
as he thrusts

Lie still while your lover grinds
you to ecstasy

a delicious chance for a man
to let his hips do the talking

As he drinks at his lover's delta,
she drinks pure air

a vibrant position that
helps the woman free herself
from shyness

A flare of excitement that will dazzle him

gentlemen,
don't be shy:
tell her how
much you
love this

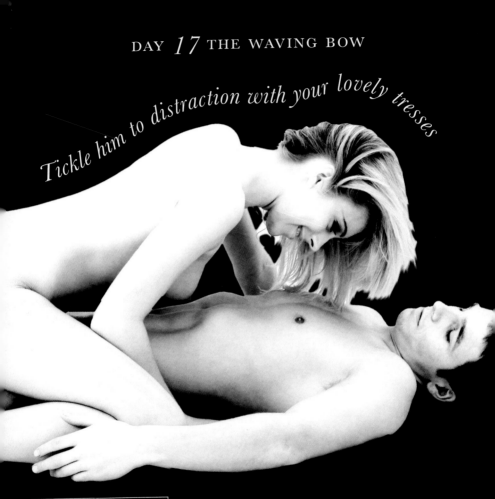

Tickle him to distraction with your lovely tresses

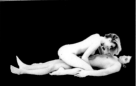

playful and exciting at the same time,
this is a charming way to seduce him

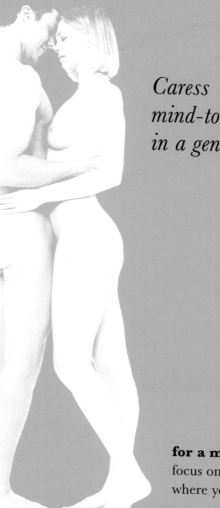

*Caress
mind-to-mind
in a gentle embrace*

for a meditative thrill,
focus only on those places
where you touch

Press together so your bodies seem almost to penetrate each other

an embrace
that can melt
without warning
into lovemaking

A naughty nip goads her into punishing you

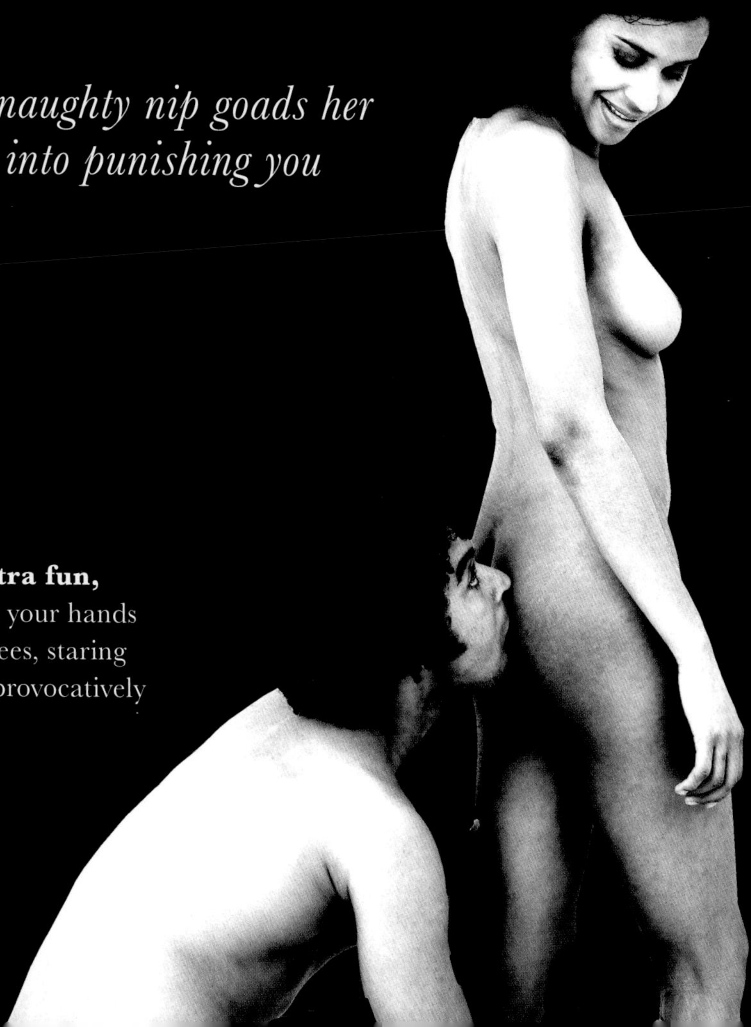

for extra fun,
stay on your hands and knees, staring at her provocatively

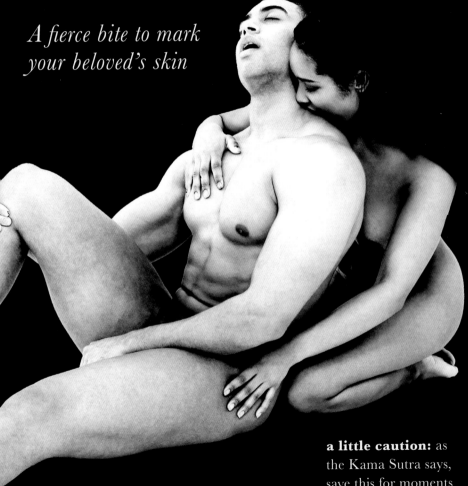

A fierce bite to mark your beloved's skin

a little caution: as the Kama Sutra says, save this for moments of intense passion

Wind and wind around
until her head spins

the Kama Sutra advises you
to probe with your nose and chin
as well as your mouth

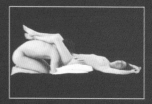

A light circle of marks on a beautiful breast

gentle but firm, a tease to bring passion to a lightning frenzy

Play together with innocent delight

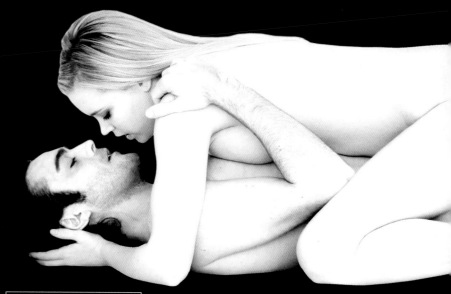

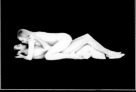

a sweet position
recommended by the
Smaradipika

Mingle and merge for infinite enjoyment

a comfortable
position for
easy entry

A turn of the hand to entangle his heart

with each downward
stroke, add a little twist over
his most sensitive point

DAY *27* THE FOLDED LILY

Pleasure her until she blooms with ecstasy

comfortable but vigorous, a favorite for loving couples

*Make your
beauty thirsty
for more*

a light lick and
suck that makes
even the shyest
woman eager

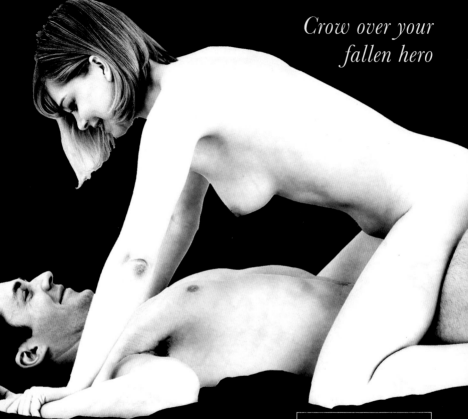

*Crow over your
fallen hero*

Vatsyayana tells a woman in
this position to laugh at him,
drunk with conquest

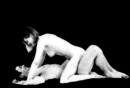

Squeeze and stroke him inside your vice

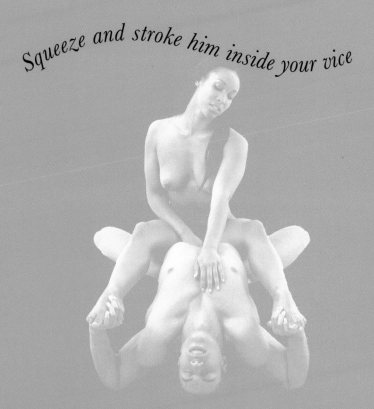

the Kama Sutra says this
takes long practice; Dr. Kegel
would say that's a fine idea

DAY *31* THE ATTENDANT

*Form a circle
of caressing,
from head to toe*

the man enjoys his
woman's tender touch
and her silky legs in
perfect ease

Cover her eyes to uncover her fantasies

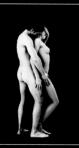

hold your beloved
secure while she
whispers her
darkest dreams

DAY *33* CHUSHITA (SUCKED)

Draw deep kisses from her well of pleasure

the Kama Sutra
suggests that you add
some nibbling as well

Tread the breathless border between pain and pleasure

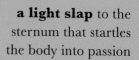

a light slap to the sternum that startles the body into passion

Decorate her with a secret memento

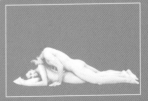

bite gently, but enough to
leave a trace she can cherish

A delectable massage for her succulent breasts

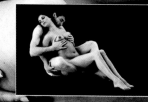

the woman rests
against her lover,
thinking of nothing
but his circling hands

Hold him hard for a moment before releasing

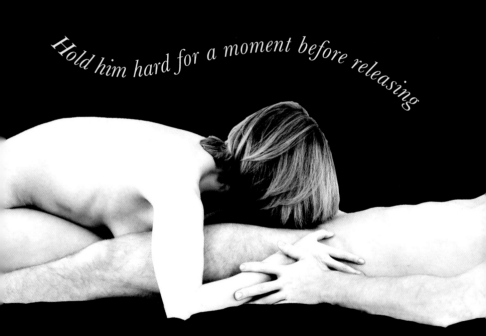

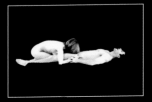

Don't forget to cover
your teeth with your lips

Rock, rock, rock with your beloved

a position that's
both fun and tender

A vigorous position that shakes the woman's body into frenzy

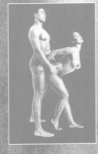

with one foot loose, clasp your lover's hips for steadiness so you can move freely

Buck underneath your beauty to scatter her wits

with his legs bent back, he can thrust with unexpected force

*A woman who can
spread herself like this
has reason to be vain*

**for those who can manage
it,** this gives a stretched,
wide-open sensation

He'll travel far for a treat like this

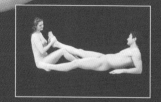

don't forget that life is a
voyage together, so do this often

Press together suddenly, shocking the breath from each other

a swift
yet tender
caress for new
lovers building
their intimacy

*Rake your mark across
your doe's flank*

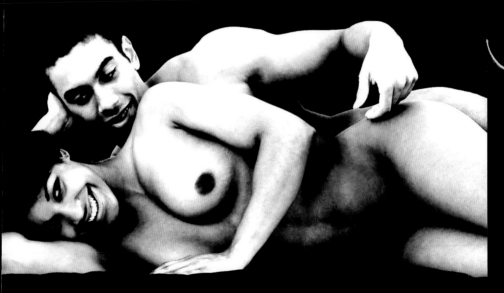

the Kama Sutra suggests
that nail play is particularly
thrilling before and after
a long separation

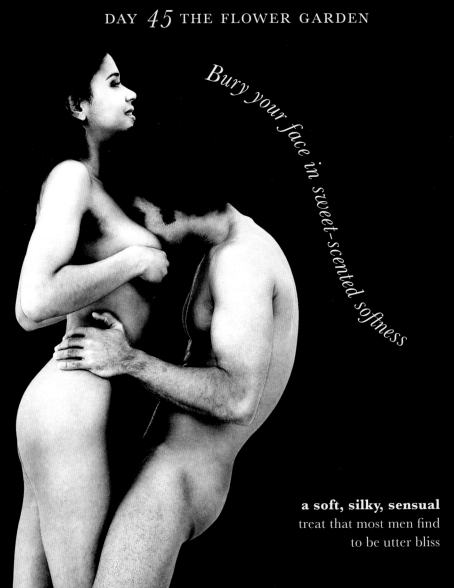

Bury your face in sweet-scented softness

a soft, silky, sensual
treat that most men find
to be utter bliss

Knead and groom your handsome prey

to make a game of it, nip
him lightly if he squirms

Twist and nestle together, freestanding like dancers

an embrace that suits both gentle and passionáte moods

*Caress belly to belly, melting
into each other*

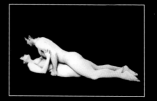

a hold that presses each
jaghana (middle part of the body)
against the other

Curl your hand into a snake-hood shape and strike

cupping the hand
cushions the impact,
so this is great for
playful swatting

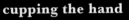

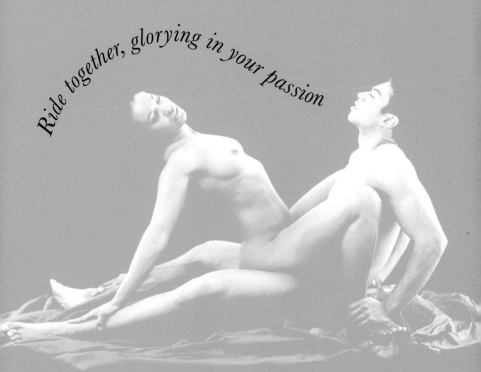

Ride together, glorying in your passion

a good grip on each other's legs gives this position a nice, secure feeling

Squirm and dance over your lover's moving mouth

men, let your woman lead the way while you honor her with your tongue

DAY *52* THE LOVER'S HEARTBEAT

As his fingers tap to the rhythm of her pulse, she feels the boundaries between them melt

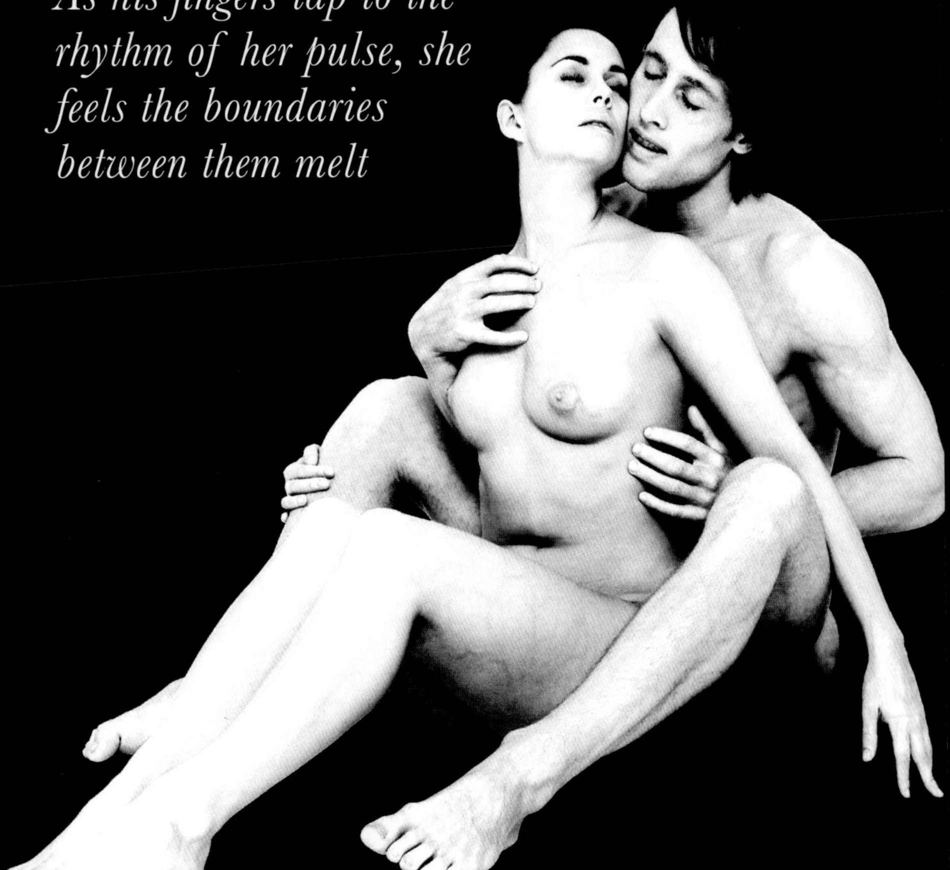

a sensual meditation
for true romantics

Catch your ankles and trap him close

holding him in place
can be thrilling at the
height of passion

DAY *54* PLUCKING THE PETALS

Tug gently at her lips to release her nectar

one that can be tried
with or without lubricant
for different sensations

Thigh to chest, relish your lover's fine flesh

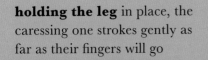

holding the leg in place, the
caressing one strokes gently as
far as their fingers will go

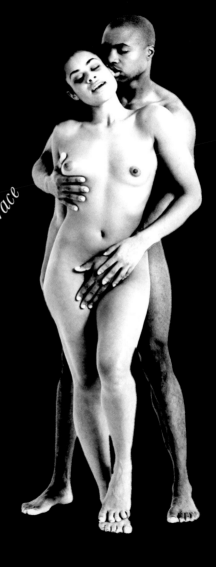

Slide into a sensuous embrace

a caress that can easily slip
into deeper pleasuring as the
lovers' hands wander

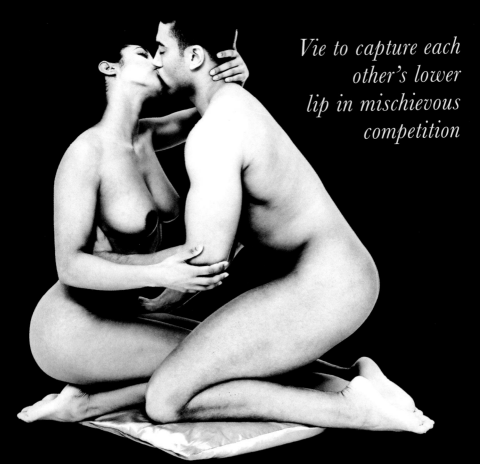

*Vie to capture each
other's lower
lip in mischievous
competition*

if you lose, Vatsyayana says to
protest that your lover cheated and you
want another chance

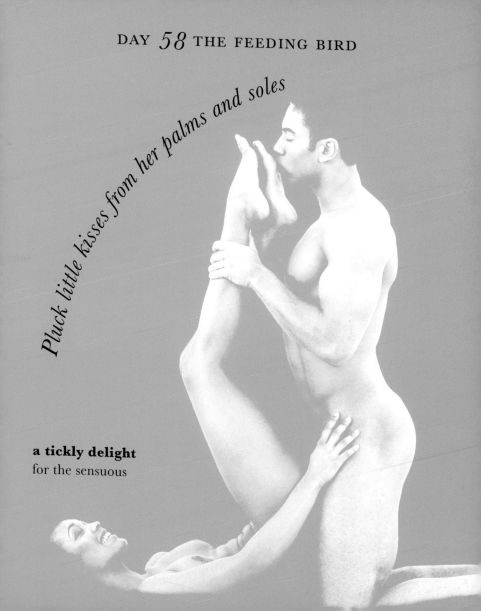

Pluck little kisses from her palms and soles

a tickly delight
for the sensuous

Draw long strokes of pleasure until he begs for release

pause a little at the end of each, so he is always on the brink of climax

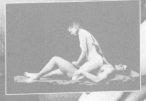

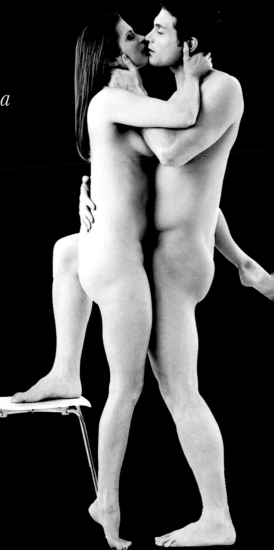

*Catch each other in a
moment of impulse*

a chair can serve
to steady you when
you're too excited
to find the bed

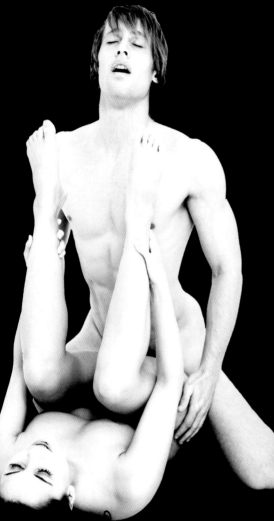

*Enter between sweet,
smooth limbs*

excellent for deep
penetration, or, if you
prefer, for anal

Primal thrusting for deep penetration

a position that tests the man's strength and awakens his virility

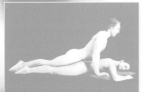

Cast away all restraint and let desire overwhelm you

a wild position for
energetic lovers

DAY 04 BAHUCHUSHITA (SUCKED HARD)

With all the force of your lips, work her to please her

she can quickly escape if the sucking becomes too much, so go at it with passion

DAY *65* THE RUDDER

Holding tight to his legs, she steers herself to climax

a chance for the man to show off his strength and flexibility

*Sweep her off her feet
and into fantasy*

men of good aim may find
themselves inside their women
before they reach the bed

Open yourselves to headlong excitement

the Kama Sutra advises the man to enter his lover gently in this position

Coax your beloved from the depths of sleep to the heights of passion

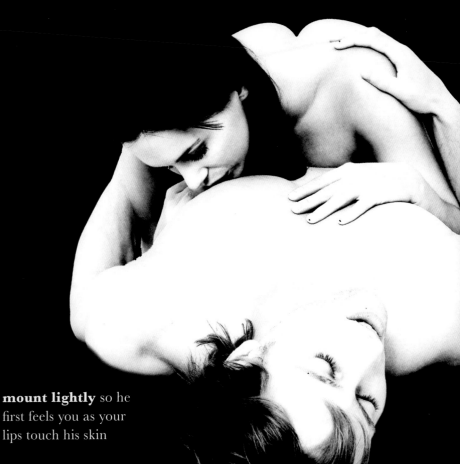

mount lightly so he first feels you as your lips touch his skin

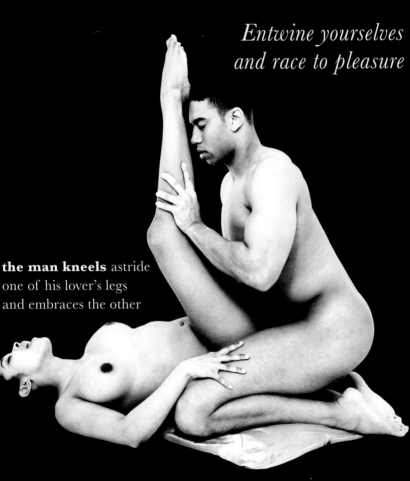

*Entwine yourselves
and race to pleasure*

the man kneels astride
one of his lover's legs
and embraces the other

Rub his tired shoulders until he drifts into sleep

a kind courtesy after a
position that wearies him

*Flick up a silky limb
for exotic enjoyment*

a lithe variant of the
standard all-fours, good
for creating interesting
pressures on him

*Give your beauty an
open-palmed slap to
feed her passion*

the Kama Sutra
reminds us that love-
blows are a matter of
taste, so be sure she's
willing before you try

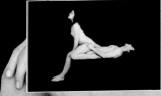

A man who so ascends his lover's body can truly delight in her shapely curves

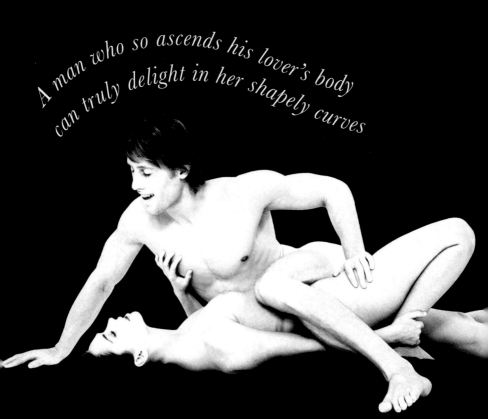

penetration may be tricky, but with some massage oil he can rub blissfully against her pretty stomach

Admire your lover's beautiful form as she pleasures you deeply

a careful woman guards her teeth with her bottom lip to protect his manhood from harm

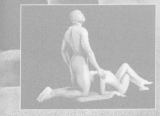

Streak little tracks in her waiting skin

the Kama Sutra calls it unchivalrous to go on a journey without leaving at least a few scratched mementos

Slide together, hands forgotten

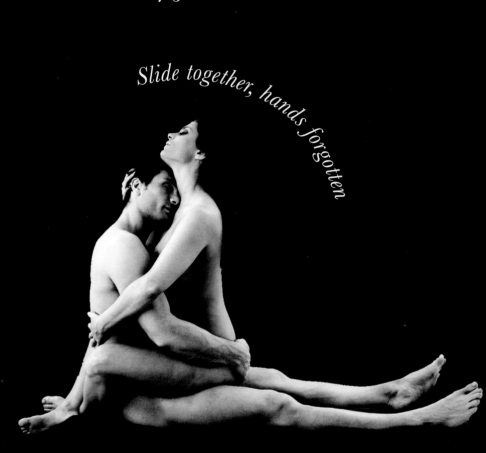

a thrilling way to
enjoy each other all over

DAY *77* THE SCULPTING CARESS

Trace the shape of your man's head as you whisper why you love his mind

pressing your body against his while you stroke unites flesh and spirit in tenderness

With all exposed, let your tongue wander freely

an earthy pleasure for
the uninhibited

*Study his secrets with your
learned fingers*

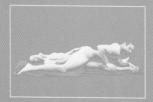

an affectionate
pose that allows
him to relax and
be explored

*Hold hard
and tight and
thrust full-speed*

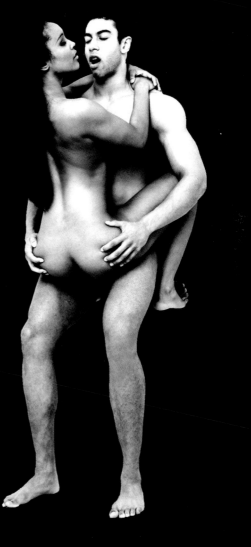

a tiring position
to sustain, so take
full advantage
and go all-out
while it lasts

Make a throne of your man and gaze haughtily down

an uncommon pose for a man: he should surrender and enjoy the novelty

*Intermingle until you can hardly
tell one from the other*

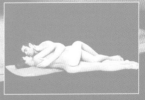

an intimate embrace
that can lead to lovemaking—
or just to love

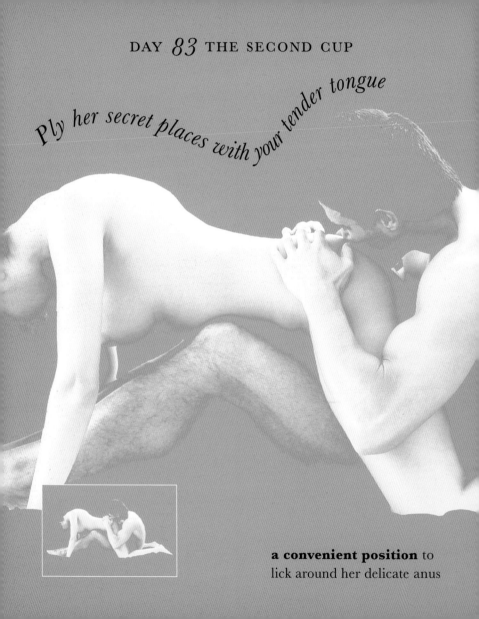

DAY *83* THE SECOND CUP

Ply her secret places with your tender tongue

a convenient position to
lick around her delicate anus

*Build up your fire with a
little support from below*

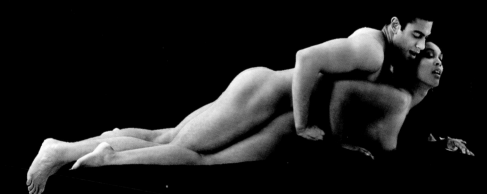

a well-placed pillow
can be just the thing to
achieve the perfect angle

Sweet-seeking lips are always a thrill

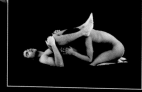

pluck lightly at his balls
until he's all in a twist
with anticipation

*Feel the warmth
and shape of each
other in blind bliss*

closing her eyes,
she explores his muscles
and bones through
pure touch

Thrust to the rhythm of the ocean until both your bodies echo with joy

a braced and bracing stance that allows for deep penetration

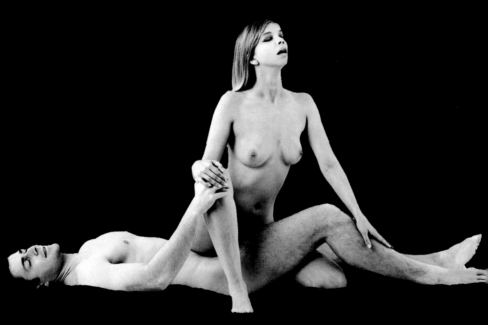

DAY *88* FEIGNING INDIFFERENCE

*He thrusts, she looks away and
pretends to ignore him*

a particularly good game
for after-argument sex

DAY *89* THE WINE PRESS

Lean deep to crush the tension out of him

thrusting can take a lot out of a man, but a
clever woman knows how to keep him refreshed

*The man's fingers
press the hope of
sweeter pleasures into
his woman's lip*

men, stroke first
what you will kiss
later and your
lover's attention
is caught

Guide each other through pressure and counterpressure in a reclining dance

a position of mutual power: the man can thrust deep while the woman can control his distance with her foot

Ply your tongue on his most secret sensitive spot

between the balls and anus is an oft-neglected treasure— give it attention and listen to him gasp

A tingling, floating break from gravity

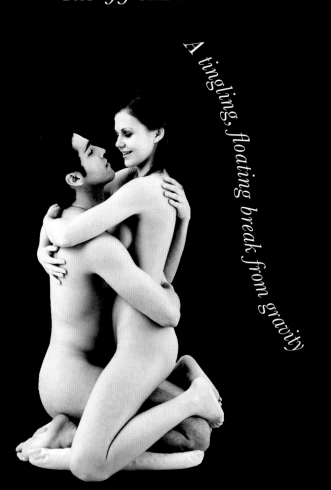

all the thrusting falls
to him here; let him
enjoy the control

Deep penetration and silken kisses play in divine counterpoint

for women who love having their toes nibbled, this is a revelation

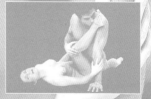

*Hold your graceful woman
and let your fingers pluck*

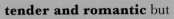

tender and romantic but
also sexy and exciting: a true
lovers' favorite

Open up your throat and take your lover in

a skill that most need to practice, but men never forget the women who master it

Gentle movements flowering into delight

a position in which to rock gently, keeping each other's comfort in mind

DAY *98* THE SPOKED WHEEL

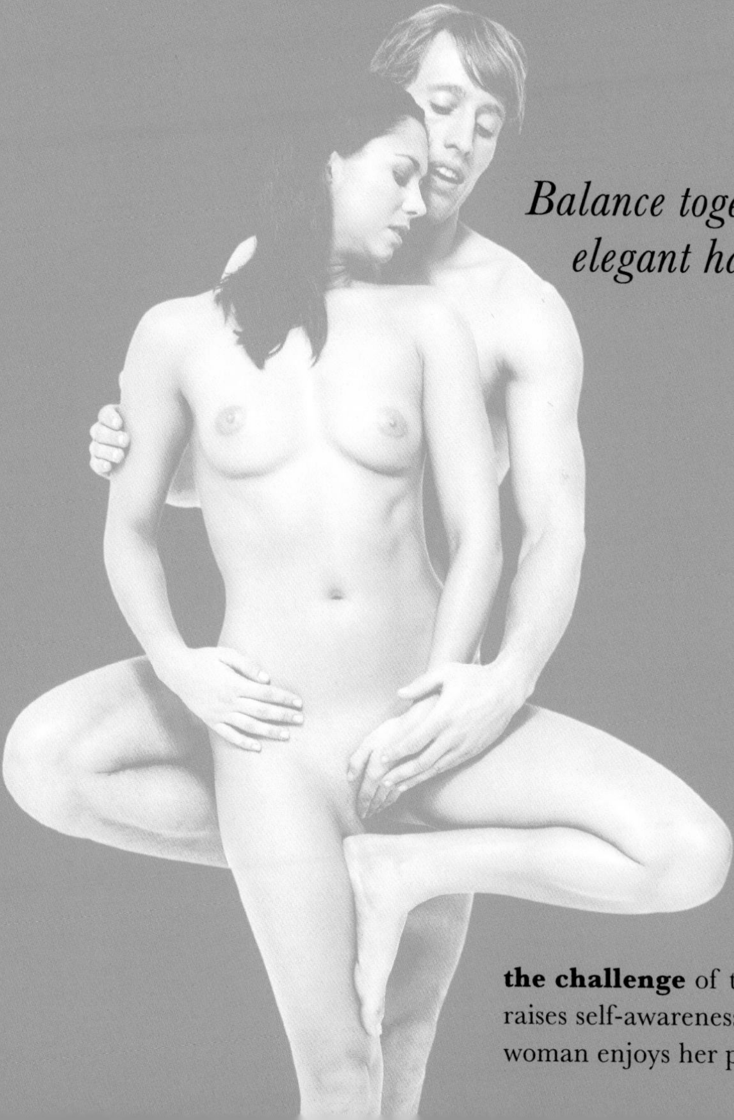

Balance together in elegant harmony

the challenge of the pose raises self-awareness as the woman enjoys her pleasuring

A cultured fellow knows when to tease

if she doesn't like having her navel tickled, you can just threaten to do it and watch her squirm

*Drift into delight on
your lover's lap*

**a pleasantly
stable** and easy
variant of the
feet-off-the-ground
position for her

Knead her delicious flesh until she rises to your touch

a man who attends to his lover's shoulders will always be welcome in her bed

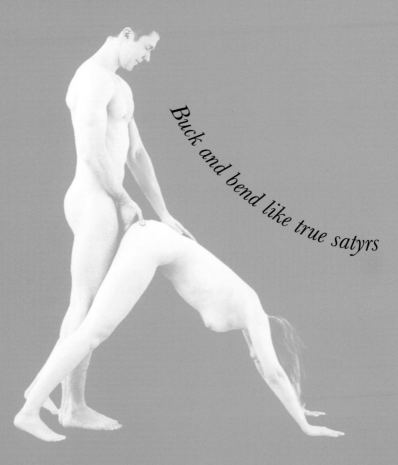

DAY *102* GOAT CONGRESS

Buck and bend like true satyrs

the upward angle allows the man a vertiginous view of his woman's back and bottom

Leap together until she chirps in delight

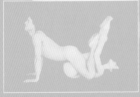

a position for playful lovers
looking to challenge their bodies

*Catch each other's lips and suck
in languorous ease*

the Kama Sutra defines this
as her kissing his upper lip
while he kisses her lower lip

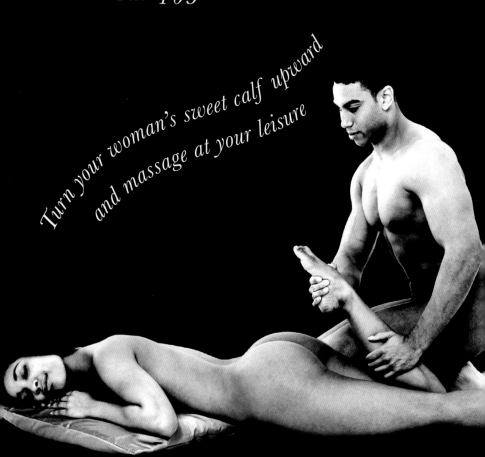

DAY *105* BENDING THE REED

Turn your woman's sweet calf upward and massage at your leisure

true relaxation for the woman that will always make her appreciate her man

*Take your
lingering, licking,
luscious time*

according to the Kama Sutra,
the Crow is so much fun that
many a courtesan abandoned
patrons who wouldn't indulge in it

Break through shyness to love

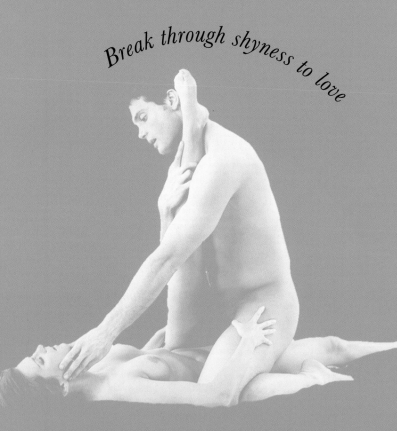

if she turns her eyes
away in unusual positions,
gently steer her face and
coax her to look at you

*A man treasuring his lover's
yoni and breasts at once
has wealth indeed*

a springy position
that allows for
deep enjoyment

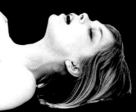

*Angle your bodies apart
to luxuriate in the cool
air on your skin*

an embrace best tried on
a soft floor for a good stable base

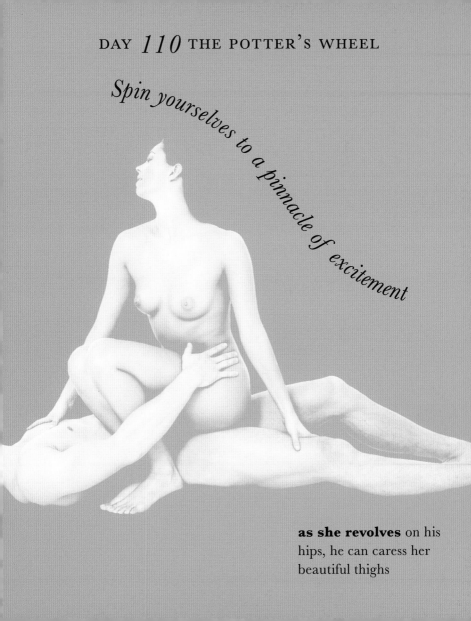

DAY *110* THE POTTER'S WHEEL

Spin yourselves to a pinnacle of excitement

as she revolves on his hips, he can caress her beautiful thighs

DAY *111* THE BENDING EMBRACE

*Press down on your beloved
and shower her
with kisses*

if the man's
hold is strong, this can
be a deeply passionate
embrace

Gazing at the man's face, his beloved kisses him to wakefulness

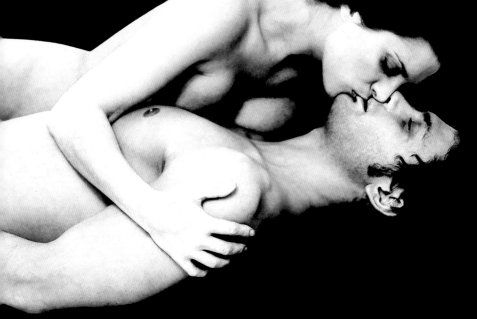

a delicious experience
that can kindle any kind of
lovemaking

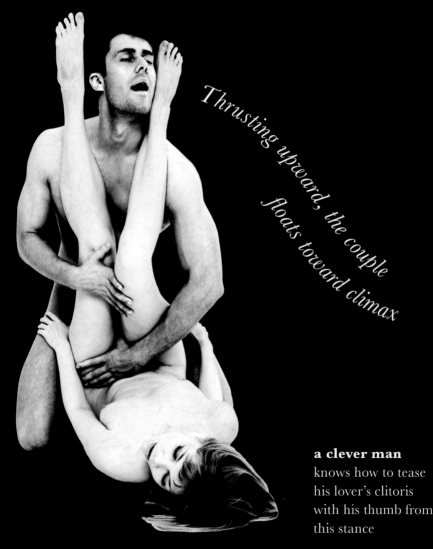

Thrusting upward, the couple floats toward climax

a clever man knows how to tease his lover's clitoris with his thumb from this stance

*Let her drift into a
dream of sensuality*

at once arousing and
soothing, this is a fine stroke for
deepening love

*Tickle him from below with
your soft-stemmed tongue*

a marvelous way to startle
him into uninhibited laughter

*A beloved woman is no burden
if her hands wander to
delicious places*

a challenge for the
man to keep steady as
his excitement builds

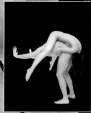

*It's easy to be overwhelmed
when you're off-kilter*

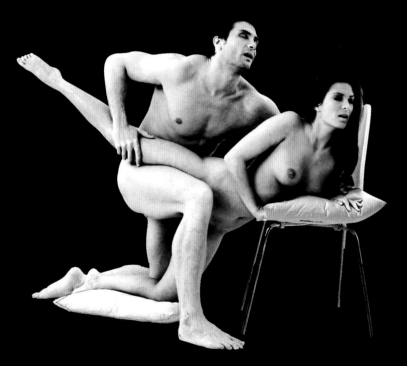

good support for elbows and knees adds
greatly to her comfort here

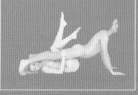

*Slither up and out—
and in again*

a tricky and roguish position for
lovers who like to laugh together

*A simple treat for the
sophisticated lover*

the Ananga Ranga
teaches that this is a
favorite with chitrini,
or artistic women

A woman of strength and vitality can draw her man down paths of endless pleasure

a position that tests the muscles, to be tried in a comfortable setting

Get his muscles and his passion all worked up

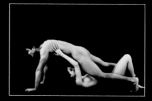

the strain of this pose can help drive the man toward an intense orgasm

Shameless admiration of his tipped-up darling

a position that lets a man show all of his vigor

Tantalize and tease a resting man with your stimulating claws

alternate massage and light scratching to drive him to distraction

*She tucks her limbs tight
as a spring shoot*

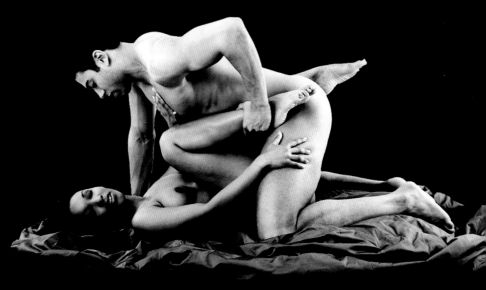

a fine position for
deep entry

With a woman's treasures right before him, a man can quest with tongue and lips

a chance to explore the delicate skin of the anus as well as the clitoris and yoni

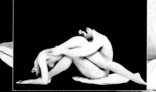

*Fly safely home into
your beloved*

an energetic
but affectionate
position that
lets pleasure
take flight

Passion distills into pure love

a tender and
wonderful caress for
the resting couple

*Even the most elegant form
bends to this temptation*

come up behind her and kiss
the back of her knee until her
legs give way

Drive forward into passionate depths

this requires a strong woman, but allows the man to thrust fast and hard

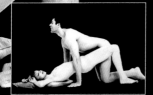

The delicate flesh of a woman's earlobe is a feast for the tender tongue

hold your lover firmly while she squirms in ecstasy

Rain one salute after another onto her satin skin

a romantic sequence that can go anywhere on a lover's body

DAY *132* TWO HANDS AT WORK

Slide up one then the other for never-pausing arousal

use lubricant for smooth, unbroken flow

DAY *133* SLIDING STRIKE

*Slip in slow and pull
out fast—a sweet
reverse rhythm*

a vigorous yet
careful stroke, good
for when she's open
and vulnerable

A rough-and-ready stance for lingering strokes

the Panchasayaka defines the
Tripod as the man holding one
of the woman's knees while his
hands caress her

Match each other limb-to-limb to ignite your tenderness

a position suited to embraces, where the man can admire his woman in all her glory

Hold your lover entirely as you penetrate her deeply

an unusual angle that lets lovers explore new thrills

*Nibble lightly until
anticipation shivers
into pleasure*

**a light, exploratory
kiss**—save your
tongue for later

*Round your lips and
kiss passionately*

hold off on the sucking
and lavish all your attention
on his sensitive underside

DAY *139* THE LIONESS

Thrust deep and let loose your primal roar

the Kama Sutra says you can choose which animal you pretend to be, so pick a great one

*A feat of balance to
show off to each other*

**if you get
comfortable,** this
allows for deep
penetration, but
clowning can be
fun too

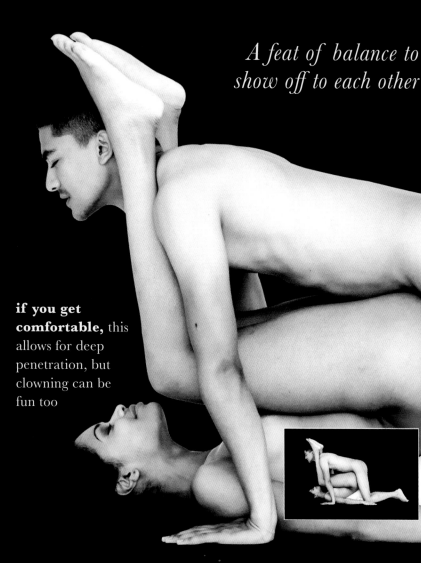

Press yourselves together in animal curiosity

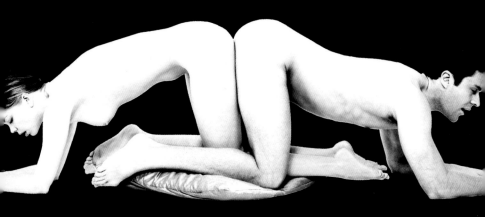

a playful embrace to explore
each other genital-to-genital

Wrap each other in languid sensuality

a comfortable position for
slow, loving congress

Nestle up behind her for a good muzzle

a fun way to get
your beauty's attention
in the morning

Furled around her lover, she grows tender

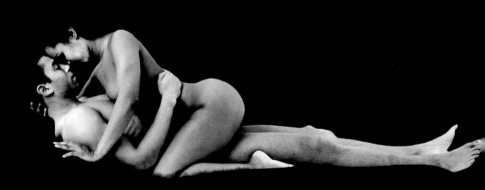

a way to fill your romance
with the joys of spring

A grinding, glorious twist

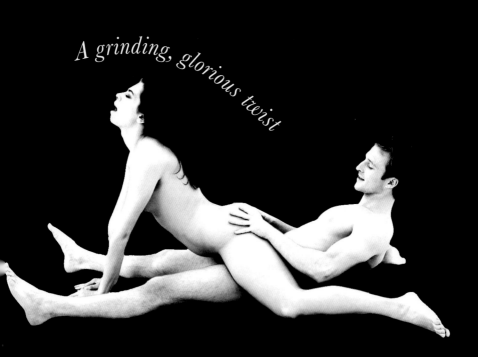

particularly good if
his erection naturally
angles downward

DAY *146* THE NESTING CROW

Let the beautiful woman mount to the heights

a comfortable variation
on an old favorite

Hold your woman's thighs and enjoy her feminine flesh

this embrace lets the man appreciate his lover's lush legs while nestling his genitals close to hers

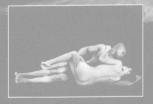

Lean against a wall as your lover grinds her hips to pleasure you both

in this posture, the man acts as an anchor while the woman controls the movement

Slide slowly up and down his jade stem, taking time to feast your senses

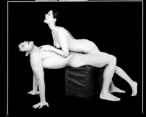

the man should have a stool to brace himself, as this position is taxing

*Tap and tease until
her body sings*

drum your fingers on her
tenderest parts in a light,
percussive rhythm

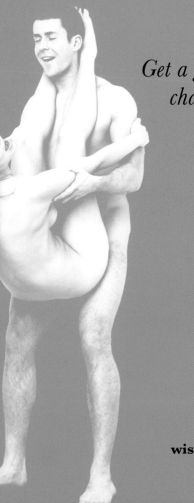

Get a good grip and challenge gravity

wisest to do this over a soft surface for your own peace of mind

No shadow can fall on pleasure this bright

the tension of keeping her leg straight tautens the woman's muscles to sculpted perfection

Swinging free in the air, the woman's joy rises above the earth

if she can keep a good grip
with her legs, his hands are
free to pleasure her

*Dig deep and slow in
her soft furrows*

he might slip out if you
try this too fast, so go at a
good measured pace

*A shivering,
sensuous thrill*

don't quite kiss:
just let your breath
tickle your lover's
stretched skin

*Wrapped lightly in her lovely legs,
he presses forward*

a position that suits
anal penetration as well

*Stretch into your
lover's lap with
regal grace*

the curve of her spine
raises her breasts
proudly against him

*A dream of
pleasure and a
dream of grace
combined*

the man should
take a steady stance
and be sure to hold
his lover securely

*Breathless anticipation before the
downward swoop*

a pose that tantalizes her desires while
impressing her with his strength

*Offer yourself up for
absolute exposure*

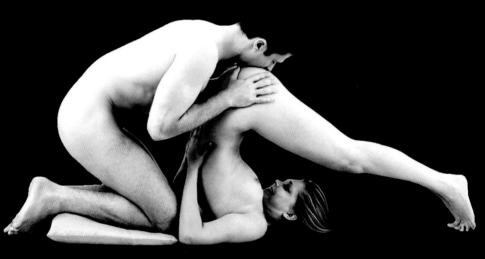

if she's limber enough to
sustain this, the rush of blood
to the head is thrilling

*Wind branching loops
of love bites around
your lover's neck
and shoulders*

the Kama Sutra
suggests pressing only
with the upper incisors

Feel the motion as you ride secure against your lover's thighs

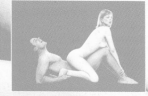

from this position, a man can admire his lover's back and bottom while enjoying the touch of her breasts

Stir his dreams with your lips

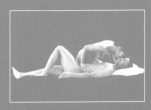

in a few minutes, he wakes up primed and passionate

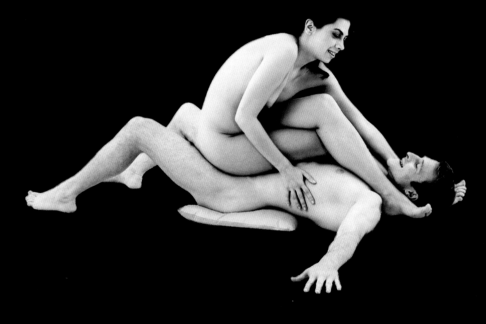

The cunning artisan unlocks her lover's desires

the crossed keys of her
feet hold his head so he
must gaze at her

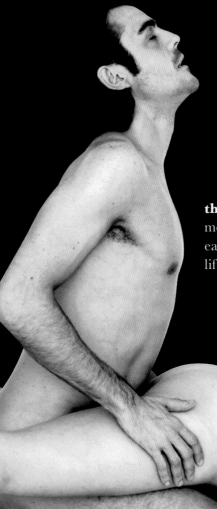

*Guide your beauty to a
freewheeling climax*

this is one of the
most natural and
easy variants of the
lifted-woman theme

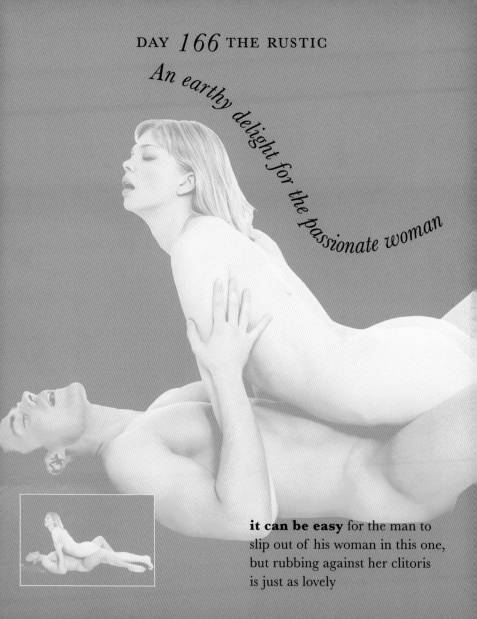

DAY *166* THE RUSTIC

An earthy delight for the passionate woman

it can be easy for the man to
slip out of his woman in this one,
but rubbing against her clitoris
is just as lovely

DAY *167* THE PULLED KNOT

Strain against each other to heighten the intensity of your connection

experienced lovers use the Pulled Knot for variation in lovemaking, moving in and out of the position

Give it a chance and see if your excitement takes wing!

of course there are easier ways to do this, but it's good to try a real challenge sometimes

Resting impaled, the woman squeezes her muscles around her lover

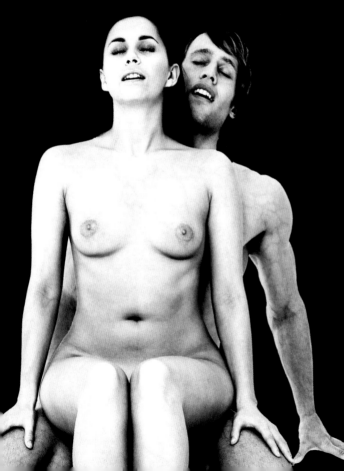

if she tires, her lover can support her by wrapping his arms around to help her balance

*Rest one atop the other and
rustle together slowly*

a sweet and tender
position for loving partners

DAY *171* PALM STRIKE

*Build up a rhythm,
making love to her skin*

pull back your fingers so
just the hard flesh of your
palm makes its impression

Arch and rub against your master

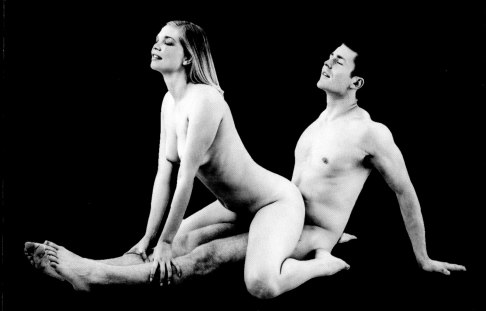

**a comfortable
stance** that allows for
affectionate role-play

*Sink in with slow,
fierce delight*

for an easier
alternative, try resting
the woman on a good,
sturdy table

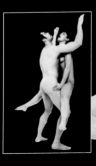

Rock to and fro against each other, keeping blissful time

challenging to the muscles but peaceful in mood, this is one for lovers who know each other well

Rock together on an ocean of pleasure

a man who braces his feet against something solid can hold his lover securely in position

Coil into curiosity

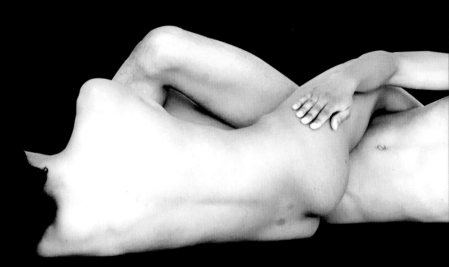

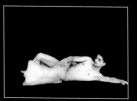

an unusual twist on rear entry
for the adventurous couple

Bolster yourself for a beautiful vista

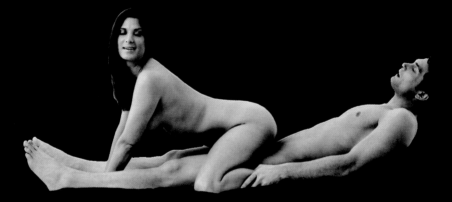

**a lovely woman's writing
back** is a sight to warm any
man, so aim for a good view

Pull your bodies taut and feel them strum against each other

when the man holds his chest still and grinds with just his hips, this is particularly exciting

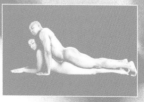

Throw your leg high around your lover and pull him to you

penetration can be a little uncertain like this, but there are few more enchanting caresses

Grind her nipples diamond-hard

her nipples can be a fast path to
passion, so pay them their due in full

*Hold fast and become
pure sensation*

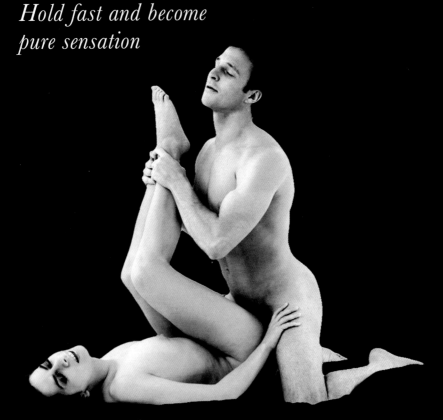

men love to gaze, but try
closing your eyes and meditating
only on what you feel

DAY *182* TUGGING THE SILK

A playful pull can awaken the helpless maiden in your woman

be sure to get a good handful, as trapping stray hairs can hurt too sharply

DAY *183* SKY FOOT

Become a firmament unto yourselves as you grow lost in passion

recommended by the
Ananga Ranga and the
Panchasayaka, this is one
for deep thrusting

*Pointing one toe,
the woman brings
elegance and spirit
to the moment*

**a position that
lets the woman**
enjoy the sensation
of her own beauty

*Be a good groom and
tend your mount*

a woman who
maintains her
lover's hardworking
muscles will reap a
handsome benefit

Pride yourself on your beautiful bust

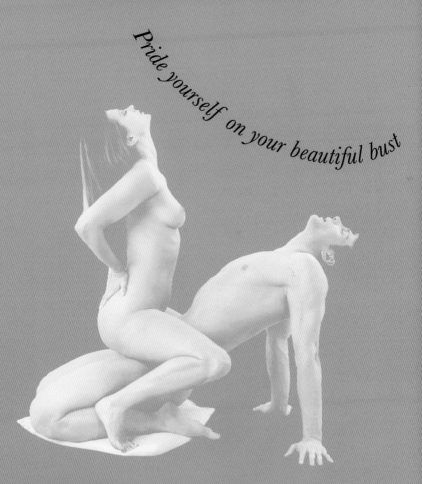

folding back the arms
like this displays her breasts
to wonderful advantage

Bend your limbs and crush together as closely as you can

a position to remember if you and your lover have only a twin bed

DAY *188* THE BEE

The woman circles her hips until both lovers are buzzing with pleasure

the Kama Sutra
advises that this
takes practice, but it
can be honey-sweet
if done well

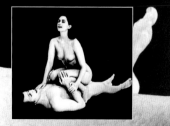

*The man's heart beats
against his princess's
dainty heels*

the Smaradipika
suggests that the man
let his hands wander
and caress

*Pin your lover in a hold
he won't wish to fight*

for extra enjoyment, grind
yourself on his helpless body

*Catch him between your
pretty feet, and he's
at your mercy*

even a light hold controls
the man; if he's a lover of feet,
this is pure heaven

Find your most daring angle

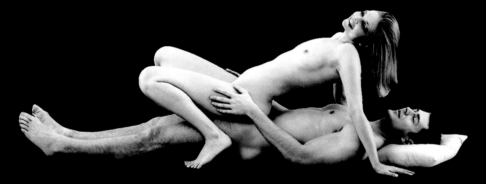

every couple has their
own fit: try leaning back
and forth to test it

Tantalize her with the heat of your mouth

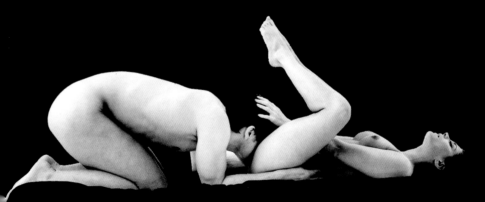

before the kissing
and licking begin, warm
her yoni until she's
frantic with impatience

A sweet and sudden embrace in which the woman clutches her man with all limbs at once

a woman enclosing her lover
like this will hold his heart as
well as his body

Plunge into a sweet tangle of flesh

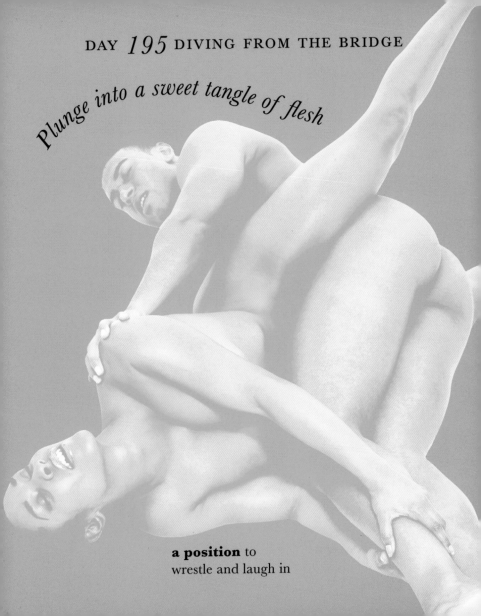

a position to
wrestle and laugh in

Stretch your woman like a bow and pluck her to climax

the man can contemplate an elegant dance melting into squirming arousal

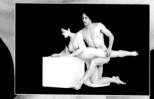

Exposed and excited, the man's whole body is within her reach

a fine position in which to take a few playful slaps at his handsome bottom

Square off for a good tussle

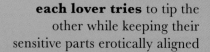

each lover tries to tip the
other while keeping their
sensitive parts erotically aligned

The woman trails a leg back to open herself to her beloved

parting her legs in this way allows her lover entry while remaining pleasantly tight

Scrape your nails lightly across your lover until his skin tingles in ecstasy

named for the sound the nails make, this is a thrilling yet gentle caress

Measure your pleasure
by squirming degrees

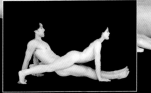

perhaps best not to
try penetration in this
pose, but excellent for
rubbing together

Make love in sweet, easy harmony

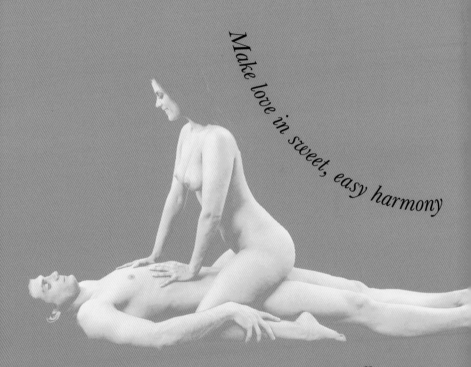

an eternally popular
position in every culture

As the man thrusts from a crouch, he drives both lovers into flight

the woman lies on a stool, or a bed if she prefers a more restful posture

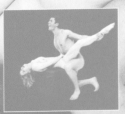

DAY *204* TWO PAINTBRUSHES

Wet your lips and work with all your craft

a challenge to sustain, but all the more artistic for that

Each lover grips the other, unable to escape and unwilling to relinquish

a game that gives each partner the thrill of both the hunter and the hunted

*Climb down to your couch in
limber playfulness*

**there's more to
lovemaking** than just
congress, so play on
each other's desires
from the outset

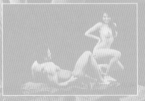

Trace your toes over his sensitive skin

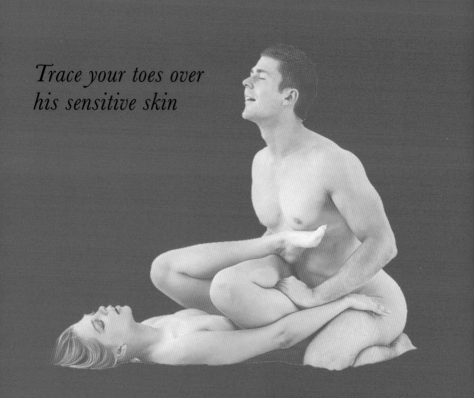

the skin of the instep is particularly satiny: let him feel just how sleek you are

Bump and bounce your way to satisfaction

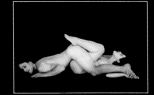

nicely comfortable for a rear-entry reverse, this is well worth a try

*Meditate together as
your flesh intermingles*

one in which
to try flexing your
love muscles in
or around
your partner

*He plays the roast, she the spit,
as they heat up together*

the Kama Sutra
suggests the woman
alternate legs, placing
one heel by his head,
then the other

Tangle yourselves tight for real passion

this position allows
for vigorous thrusting
while still feeling
friendly and tender

DAY *212* THE DEER

*Rut together
through the wild
autumn nights*

the man thrusts and
the woman swings to and
fro on her hands

Flick firm against his sensitive flesh

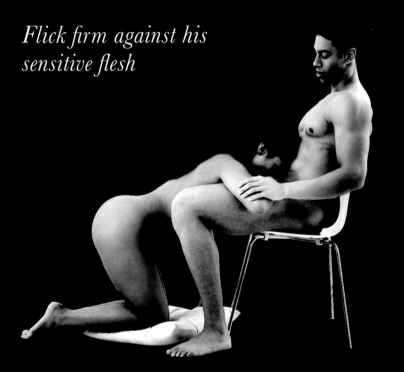

a lively variation on regular
sucking in which her tongue
delivers hard licks against his glans

DAY *214* POLISHING THE JEWEL

As you rock together, the motion of his thumb lights her up with desire

a loving man attends to his woman's clitoris during congress

*Find his flow by touch as you press
your body blindly against him*

an unusual position that
allows the man caresses from
both sides at once

She dozes in perfect innocence as he creeps up to pleasure them both

a game in which the woman feigns sleep — making sure she's coyly positioned on the bed before he enters the room

*Delicious pleasure for the
love-hungry couple*

flick your tongue
teasingly between her
toes before sucking them

Strike deep and electrifying

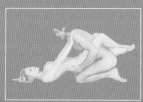

**there's nothing
like hard,** rapid
thrusts to make a
woman cry out

DAY *219* THE LANDED ARROW

As gravity draws his blood down, she works to draw it up

a challenging and submissive posture for the man, calling for strength from both lovers

Keep sliding one leg over the other for a slippery, resonant rhythm

the woman crosses and recrosses her legs to roll herself against his hand

DAY *221* LOVE'S WHEEL

Rotate your hips until your woman is dizzy with desire

this can be done by a man either
sitting or kneeling – a favorite with
passionate women

DAY *222* THE SEESAW

*Enjoy the playful
give-and-take
of new love*

a chance to refresh your
intimacy, no matter how long
you've been together

Pit your legs against each other—until you both win

a tussle of thighs that heightens the excitement of congress

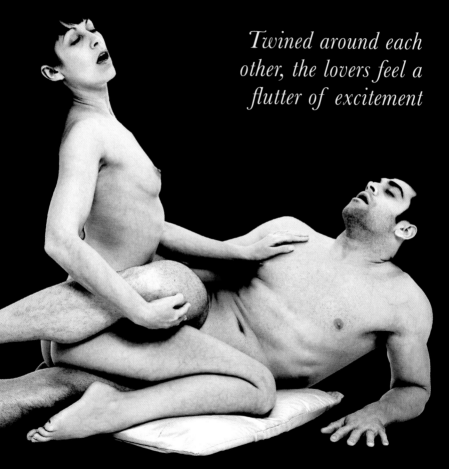

Twined around each other, the lovers feel a flutter of excitement

a position in which to rub together rather than attempt penetration, but none the worse for that

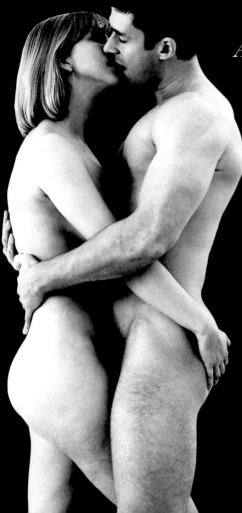

A tilted angle for long, slow exploration

sometimes it's good to get back to basics and enjoy true simplicity

Kiss your beloved as her arousal soars

an easy and delightful position
that lets the woman pleasure
herself and him at the same time

Begin the oral pleasure far from the central prize

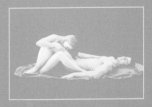

**working up the
sensitive** insides of his
thighs can leave a man
breathless and eager

Legs spiraling out like sunrays, the lovers heat each other's passion

a demanding position, especially if you attempt penetration, but a good way to enjoy feeling your lover's muscles strain

Rise and dive into joy

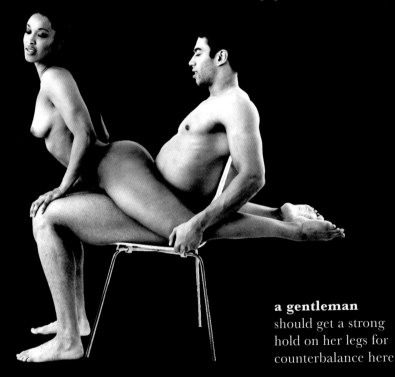

a gentleman
should get a strong
hold on her legs for
counterbalance here

Scale peaks of pleasure against your lover's virile body

try this sliding against each other's oiled skin for a non-penetrative thrill

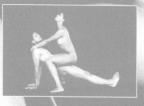

His shivering tongue deepens the tremors in her

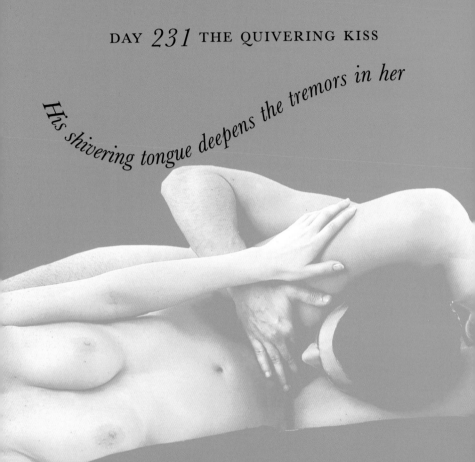

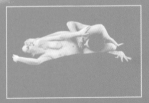

the Kama Sutra
suggests he pinch her lips
together before lavishing
them with delicate kisses

Shake your lover with the strength of your hips

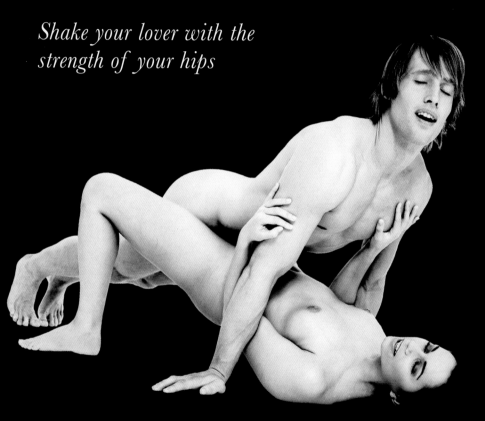

a woman rising hard against her lover challenges and matches him thrust for thrust

Tranquil as a forest floor, relax and enjoy the unusual angle

a peaceful and affectionate pose for lovers who can share comfortable silence

Rest together and let your sensations merge

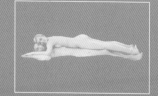

a warm, cozy full-body caress
for tender moments

DAY *235* THE JUGGLER

*Bring out your
inner circus star*

to achieve this, she
begins with a handstand
and then leans back as
he holds her

*Waken your beloved by
gently entering her body*

a game only for lovers long
acquainted—best to ask in
advance if she likes the idea

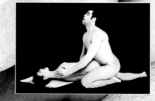

*A tantalizing approach
from behind when she
cannot go forward*

a skilled man
can coax his lover's
legs apart with
hand and member
working together

*Enter her archway with
the tip of your tongue
before licking deep*

the Kama Sutra
recommends the
lover "worship
vigorously" here

Flow into her undulating depths

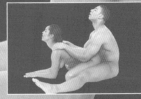

a position in which the woman controls most of the movement, as the man's legs hold his hips still

Bask together, kissing and stroking at will

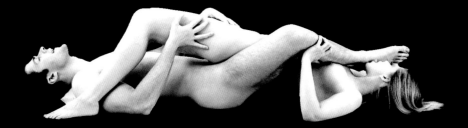

a meditative pose for lovers
delaying full congress

Dance up toward his manhood—then teasingly away

a sensual tickle for women who know how to make a man wait

Rise together to sharpen your appetites

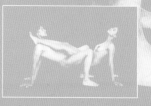

more a sexercise than a position for penetration, but excellent for foreplay

*True animal joy for
the unashamedly lusty*

a Kama Sutra classic—
trying for the legs, but
wonderful for deep
penetration

*Prepare her for a challenge
with some soft work*

those lovely thighs stretch and strain
in many positions; lavishing some care
on them can make all the difference

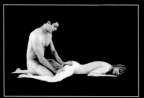

DAY *245* SPLITTING A LOG

Pull her legs as wide as they will go and ply her with full force

a favorite for men
who love to feel their
dominance

Shape the words against his waiting lips

a guessing game for lovers, with only the movement of her mouth to clue him in as to what she wants next

Pull each other close in burning passion

the Panchasayaka says that in this position the loins leap together with a sound like the flapping of elephant ears!

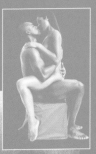

*Drift away into
deep delight*

her legs hang
in the air and
her body rocks
with the motion
of his thrusts

Don't speak—just let your expressions dance together

the power of an unbroken glance can't be overstated: spend five full minutes moving each other wordlessly

*A rush of blood dizzies
the lovely woman*

for an extra thrill,
hang your head low
enough that your breathing
constricts—as long as he keeps
your safety in mind

Keep yourselves in suspense

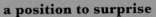

a position to surprise
and confuse our
expectations, charming for
playful moments

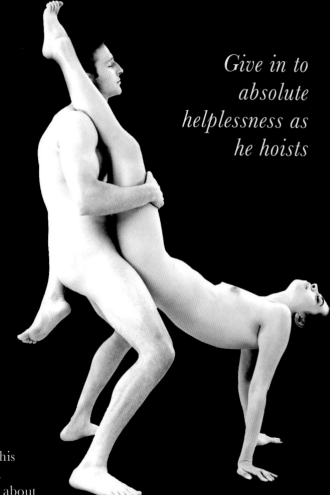

Give in to absolute helplessness as he hoists

for a man who loves to glory in his strength, this is a position to boast about

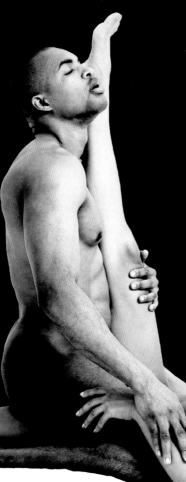

He may thrust deep, but only so far as her poised feet allow

a position in which control can shift in a moment

Let pleasure lap you as you ebb and flow together

penetration here can depend on the couple having compatibly angled genitals, but it's lovely as an embrace too

Send shivers down her spine

rake the nails very gently
across her sensitive scalp—
the resulting chills can be
surprisingly intense

Rub back and forth on his member until he gasps with desire

a wonderful double delight for him: the pleasure of her touch and the sight of her graceful movements

Trace delicate patterns of beauty across each other's backs

the contrast between the light fingers and the warm pressing of hips can be delectable

A swift, hard in-and-out that draws a cry from the most languid woman

a thrust the Kama Sutra describes as a complete withdrawal followed by a deep strike to the womb

A woman extends herself to play sacrifice for her beloved

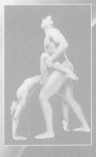

one for true gymnasts, but a fine feat if you can manage it

*Squeeze him breathless
within and without*

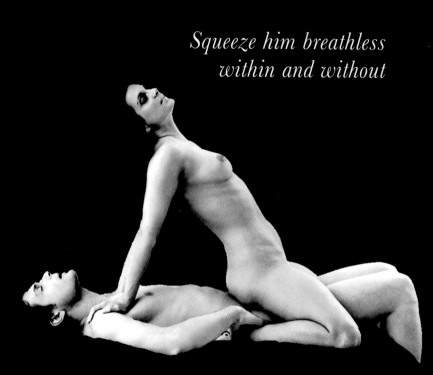

leaning back, she rests
her weight on his shoulders
for an extra frisson

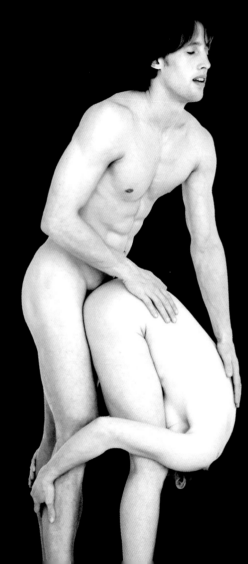

Tucked tight, ready for great pleasure to grow

a useful rear-entry position for creating a tight grip

Lift up a leg like a purring kitten and let your lover's energy refresh you

a good way to get an unusual angle, and an extra pleasure for a man who loves his woman's beautiful legs

DAY *263* PIDITAKA (PRESSING)

Sink in and push to the very depths

a love stroke the Kama Sutra
suggests for variety; if your
woman is shallow inside, be gentle

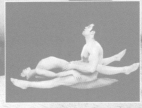

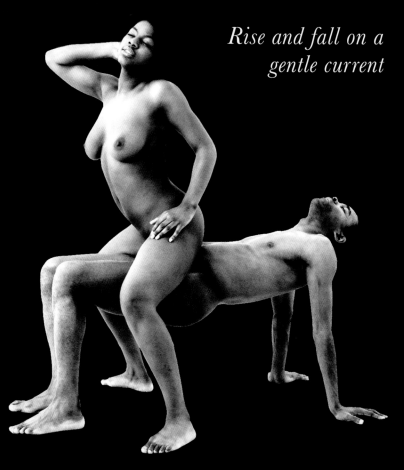

*Rise and fall on a
gentle current*

for the less athletic, add
the support of a stool or two

A yummy, yogic classic

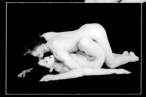

the Lotus—her legs crossed one above the other—is one of the Kama Sutra's most famous positions

*Secure your limbs
together and rock, as
carefree as children*

an energetic rise-and-fall
game to stimulate the body

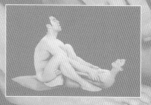

DAY *267* THE PRANCING DOE

*Leap against
your stag's
virile body*

an embrace that can
become passionate
lovemaking in an instant

Women, bend the proud male to your will

a comfortable position for the man who is ready to surrender

Twist to cast a flirtatious glance even in congress

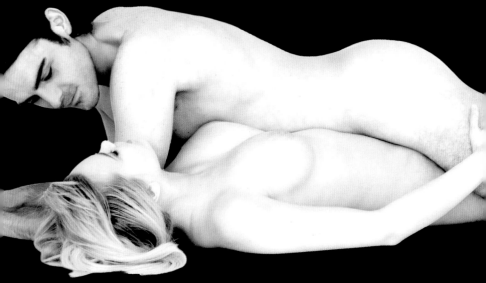

a fun variation
to liven up more
conventional sex

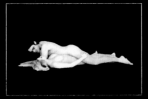

Enthrone yourself unexpectedly

a mischievous way to start
the seduction—give him a
royal surprise

Wrapped in her beauty,
the man knows delight
from head to toe

a strong man
and a small
woman work
best for this

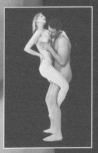

Rotate within the cave of her thighs until she cries aloud

a natural position
with a twisting thrust,
bringing out the
primal self

*Enclosed but moving
freely, the man
can thrust with
all his vitality*

pulling him closer,
the woman is
penetrated to the core

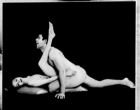

*Tuck up tight to give
him a squeeze*

there's nothing like a firm
inner grip, so roll yourself into
a ball and see what happens

Nest down on a table and feel the joys of spring

with steady furniture, the man can put real vigor into this

*Shelter between her legs
and whisper together*

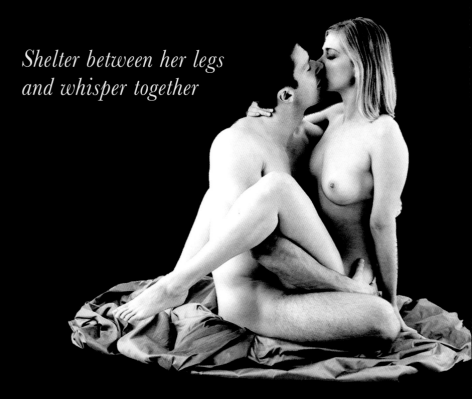

a sensual way to cuddle up
for long, sweet kisses

Sweep to and fro until you both flutter into climax

by bracing her arms both backward and forward, the woman can steady herself for long thrusts

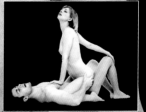

*Powered by your thrusting
legs, leap joyfully together*

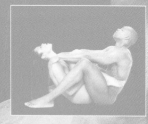

an energetic position, but
be careful not to slip apart

*Cast aside your
inhibitions and slip
straight into each other*

**one that lets
the man** feel
like a true
warrior

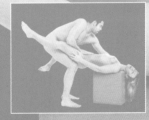

*Sweeten the moment with
a careful turn south*

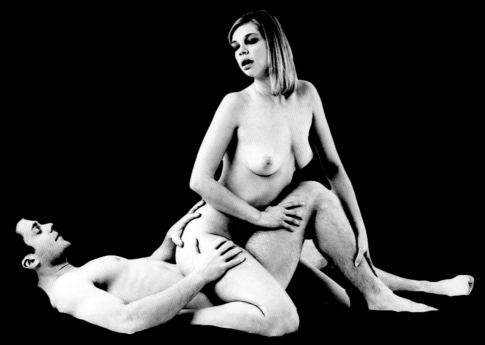

the trick is to revolve from
facing his head to facing his
feet without slipping apart

A line of delicate kisses across her dainty collarbone

for lovers looking to woo gently, this is an enchanting way to begin

Sway as in a gentle breeze

for the man,
a fine position in
which to lie back
and luxuriate in the
balmy moment

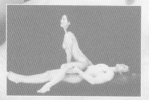

Enter your beloved freely

a stable and comfortable variant of the wide-open poses

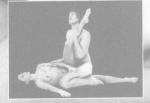

Each lover opens their lungs and inhales in the dizzy moment

a challenge for the muscles that wakes up the whole body

A lunging, plunging, flying thrill

as long as her grip
holds out, she frees
him to put all his
energy into thrusting

Creep across your resting lover with a sensuous slither

a good position
for lovers' talk
and teasing

An unexpected tickle for the tiger

women, twine a leg back
and stroke your lover's back

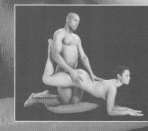

*Play a double chord
of pleasure*

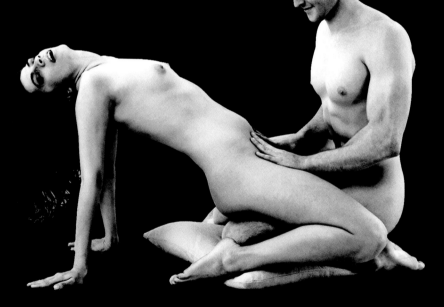

the thoughtful lover tends
to his beauty's clitoris with
a musician's skill

*Cast her down
and mold her limbs
to yours*

**a passionate
tumble** that allows
a change of positions
mid-flow

Profound abandon for the man as his beauty balances

this requires an acrobatic woman, but there's much fun to be had in trying

*Let your body be a lesson
for your lover to read*

make love without
speaking, with only
your senses for a guide

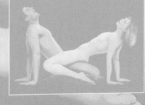

Strike wildly in all directions

the **Kama Sutra** describes this thrust as "like a bull tossing his horns"

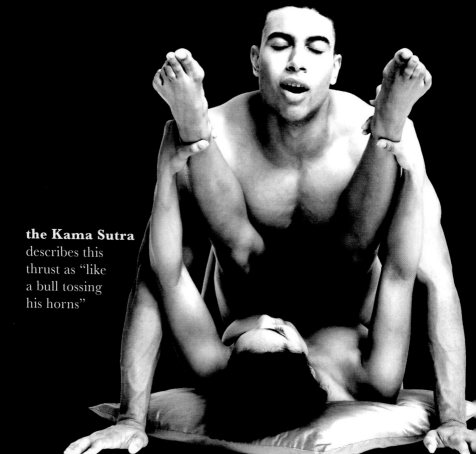

Stretch to the sky while his fingers stray to the depths

a delectable embrace
to whet the appetite

Let a stool take the weight off your minds

propping yourselves up in this position lets you think of nothing but each other

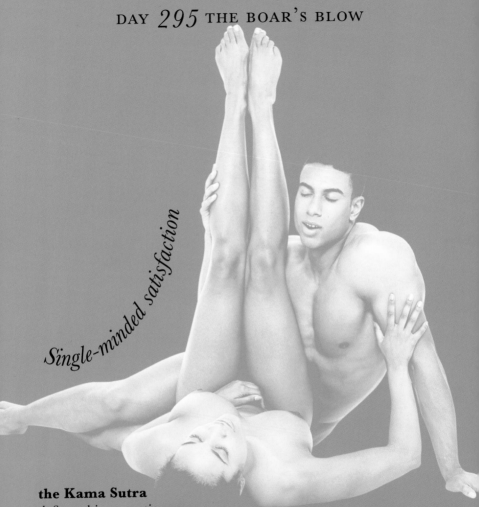

Single-minded satisfaction

the Kama Sutra
defines this as continuous
pressure on one side of a
woman's yoni

*Let yourself be pierced
with pleasure*

the Ratikallolini suggests the
woman raise one foot to her own
heart, but his chest is just as good
for the less gymnastic woman

The lightest touch can be the sweetest

**stroke ever so
gently** up and down
your beloved's skin

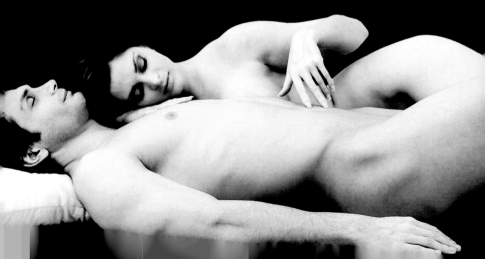

Come out of your shell ...
or let him into yours

the woman trusts her
balance entirely to her lover
and thinks only of her desire

*Stretch your body taut for
your man's excitement*

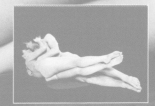

more of an embrace than a
sex position, but a wonderful way
to show off a woman's physique

Tantalize yourselves with his rising virility

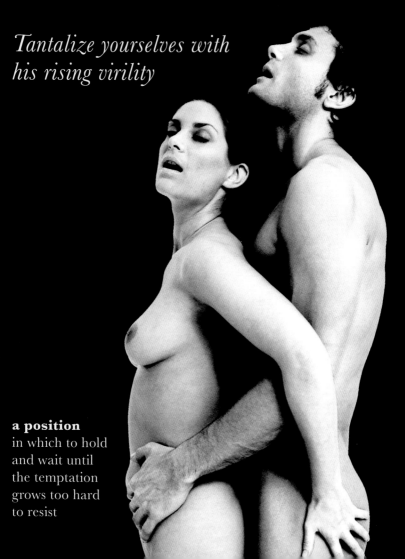

a position
in which to hold
and wait until
the temptation
grows too hard
to resist

DAY *301* THE CLIMBING MONKEY

Scamper into reckless mischief

a position
that requires a
willowy woman, but
tremendous fun if it
suits your body type

DAY *302* HALF-WRAPPED

Enclose him with a single, sinuous limb

a great deep-entry
position that's not too
limb-bendingly yogic

Pleasure yourself openly as he thrusts

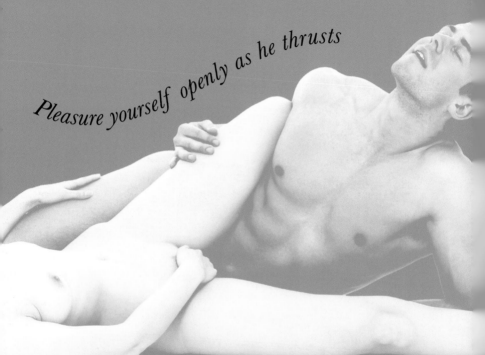

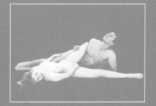

a gymnastic position that allows each lover to focus on their own excitement

Slide along a
dazzling expanse

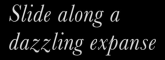

the woman who can achieve
this will be admired as a
goddess by her lover

*Rise for breath amidst
the flow of your ecstasy*

a pose the woman can
assume for relaxation
during lovemaking

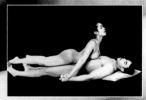

A strong man absolutely at his woman's service

a strain on all but the mightiest of thighs, but you can always move to a chair if he tires

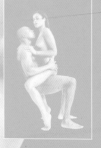

*Steal her away
from routine*

a fun way to grab
your woman's attention
and start a sexy game

Find your way and win true glory!

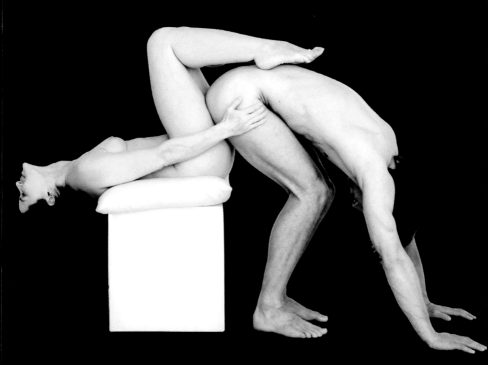

undoubtedly not the easiest angle, but a lot of fun can be had in the attempt

*Meld together and move
in perfect harmony*

a charming game
to deepen intimacy

*She lifts and
lays open her
whole body for
her beloved*

**a tender-
hearted man**
can please her
with his hand at
the same time

*Hold her safe
for the journey
into climax*

**a loving and
relaxing** position
for those times
when she deserves
all his attention

Strike down sharp

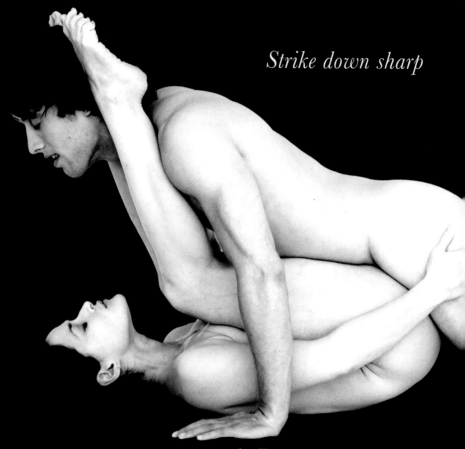

the Kama Sutra describes this
as a good stroke to add
spontaneity to your lovemaking

Raise yourself up to be your beauty's couch

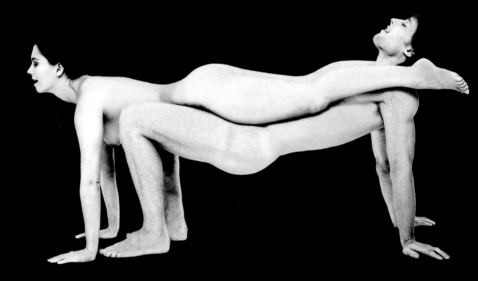

unwise to attempt penetration
here, but fine for waking up the
vigor and impressing your woman

*No man will forget
the silken delights of
his woman's skin*

**with some
lubrication,** this
is a sweet treat for
those days when
you don't want
penetration

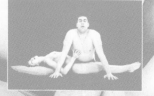

Hurl yourself into ecstasy

a gymnastic trick in
which the fear of falling
heightens the arousal

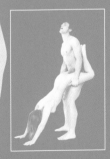

Kick up your heels and enjoy the moment

with support from a strong man, she can enjoy a moment of pure abandon

Grind and grin with your
legs all twined together

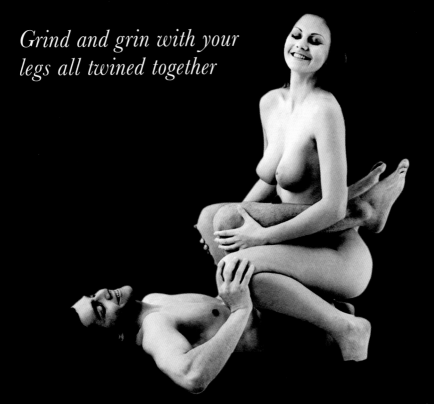

a bouncy position
that lets each partner
contribute some
flexible fun

Throw your woman back in your arms and shower burning kisses on her breast

a passionate move to sweep a woman off her feet

Meet each other's gaze in an unexpected intimacy

if you can't achieve penetration in this position, you can still enjoy the slippery fun of it

Hold steady and rub a symphony of anticipation

rather than going straight for penetration, thrust on her outer lips until you're well and truly ready

Sink with a sigh as he admires
your flowering beauty

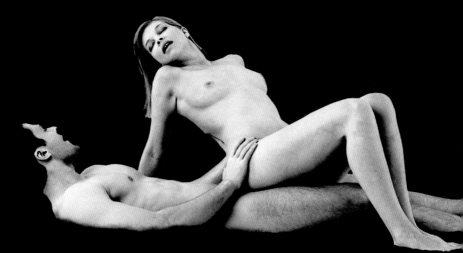

a sensuous way to
change positions and
move into a new embrace

Caress him with your feet and hands working in harmony

the Ratikallolini calls this position a way to ecstasy

Press your thighs around her so hard she gasps

a device most charming to the woman, according to the Smaradipika

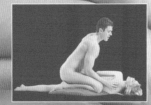

*Lean up against your man
and slide happily*

a sensuous way
for her to start the
love play

DAY *325* THE SOLDIER'S EMBRACE

Grab your chance, bed or not

an energetic position, useful for when you just have to have each other right now

Bounce in your lover's arms, a merry burden

she can be supported
with a table if need be, but
it's fun to try freestanding

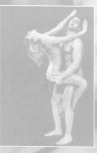

DAY *327* THE INVISIBLE TRAP

With his legs tilting her, she must move at his chosen pace

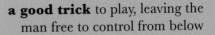

a good trick to play, leaving the man free to control from below

Rest your lips where her lifeblood beats

a deeply romantic
moment as you honor the
life in your beloved

Cling close and let your intimacy grow

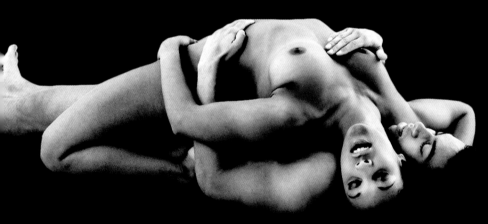

an elastic and
intimate embrace for
meditative moments

The woman sways, entirely at her man's mercy

not for beginners; there's always something new to learn in the Kama Sutra

Please her, but keep her from falling, like a true gentleman

the man shows his love by balancing his desire to caress with his pledge to keep her safe

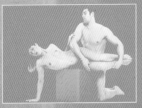

Rise from the bed as one

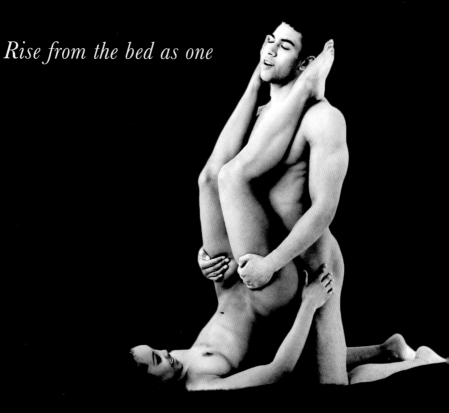

a passionate position,
calling for the lovers to
combine their strength

Call your beloved from rest with a playful breeze

a teasing, tingly way
to begin your seduction

*Get ready to be submerged
in pleasure*

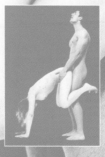

a playful and challenging
position, best tried over a
soft surface

*Prove yourselves limber
enough to rotate without
losing the connection*

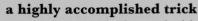

a highly accomplished trick
that must be learned with
careful practice

Wrestle hand-to-hand as your hips play a deeper game

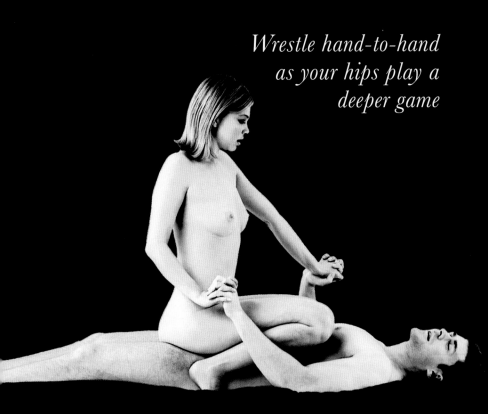

add a playful contest to heighten the thrill

Wind yourself in comfort around his strong flanks

the Kama Sutra
suggests she crosses
her legs under his
chin, but this is an
easier variant for
most people

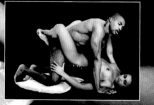

Her limbs rise and fall to the rhythm of his thrusting

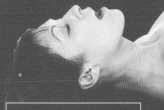

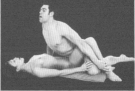

a slow, gentle twining, which the Ratimanjari compares to the sway of the fragrant jasmine plant

Trace a fingertip for his love to follow

a tender, tantalizing caress for lovers prolonging the anticipation

Wind your limbs in tangling confusion

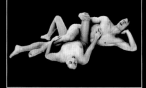

**get good and
twisted** together until
you're hardly sure
whose body is whose

Sometimes the bedroom is just too far away

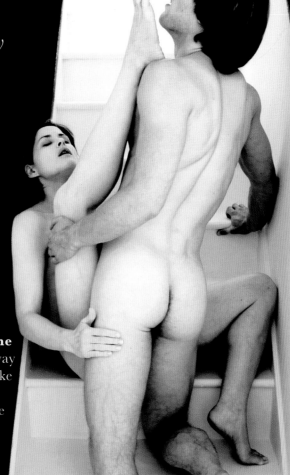

bending one leg all the way up helps make use of the limited space

*Thrust and breathe
together in perfect unison*

a sexual meditation that
combines vigorous movement
and intense self-awareness

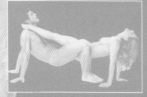

DAY *343* THE STRIDING FOX

Make a wild territory of your bed

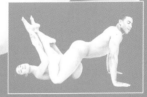

if the woman can
maintain her position, this
is surprisingly comfortable
for the man

Spring and swing, but don't let her slip away

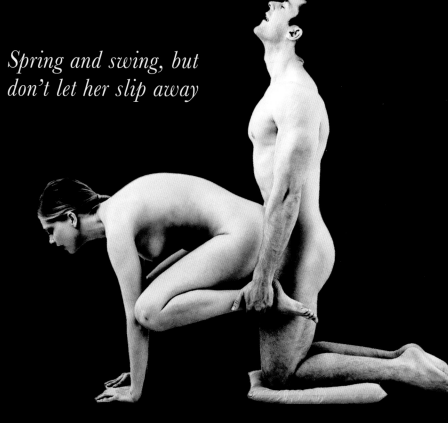

a gymnastic pose where the bounce is half the fun

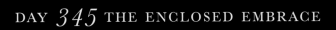

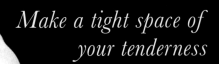

Make a tight space of your tenderness

press close up against
each other's naked skin

*Lean back on his legs
for some instant delight*

an intimate position in
which he can give her lovely
clitoris lots of attention

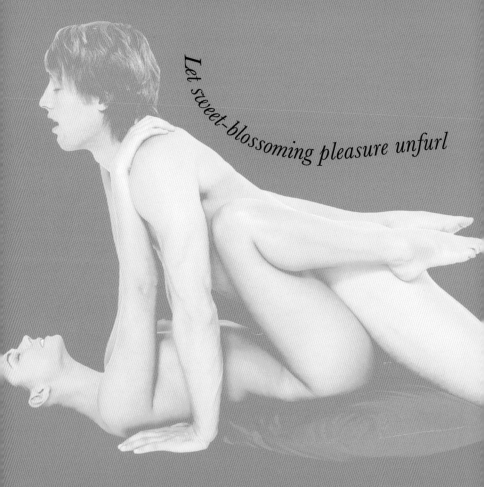

DAY *347* THE FLOWER IN BLOOM

Let sweet-blossoming pleasure unfurl

a simple position for
the passionate couple

Meet each other in the air

a man who lifts his woman
right off her feet will win
her true admiration

Drum a rhythm on your beauty with hands and hips

a gentleman should lift some of his weight off her as he pulls back for another thrust

*Tumble into a flurry
of passion*

an unusual chance for
the man to experience
upside-down delights

DAY *351* CUTTING THE ORANGE

Split open her legs and dig in deep

the unusual feeling of
sideways entry can refresh
even a familiar passion

DAY *352* THE MAN SURRENDERED

Spread and balanced, he must await his woman's pleasure

this can be done on a bed for comfort, but a stool increases his suspense

Tease with just the tip of his member

the angle makes deep penetration almost impossible, forcing the couple to partake of daintier stimulation

Squeezing, squashing sensuality

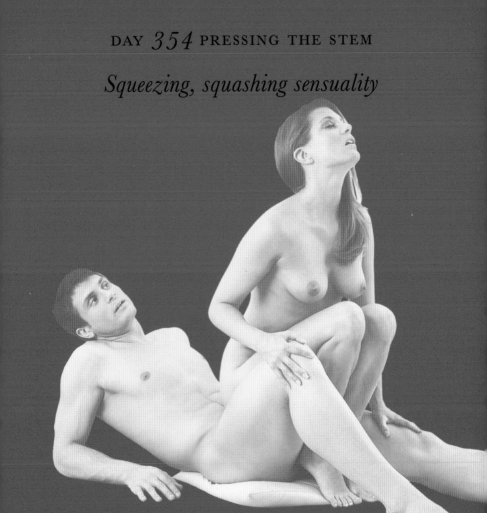

particularly good for
couples where he's a small
fit for her, as the position
tightens around him

Rise together,
inextricably entwined

fit your limbs
together in a
perfect interlace

*Pleasure her until
her limbs uncurl*

an affectionate position
for couples deeply in love

*Bend and rotate her
hips for delicious depths*

**with the
woman**
comfortable on
her back, the
man can move
her hips easily

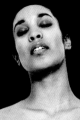

*He lies helpless
as his beauty
enjoys him*

for women who like
to take control, this is
a great way to put
him at your mercy

Kneel at her shrine for a blissful blessing

with one knee poised and one leg braced, the man can thrust with all his energy

Hold her safe while you take your gentle pleasure

a lovely sleepy embrace for
late-night intimacies

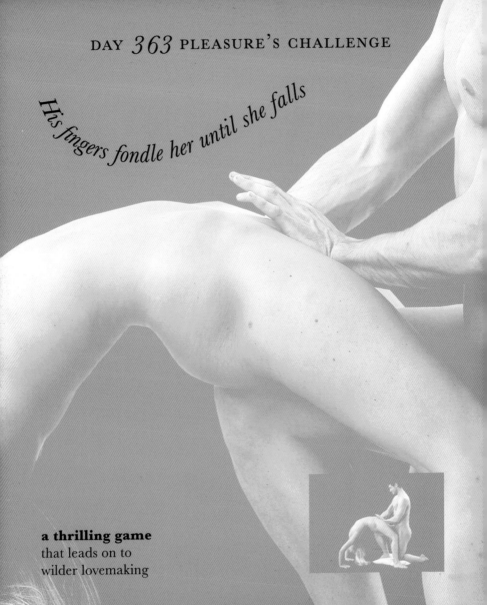

His fingers fondle her until she falls

a thrilling game
that leads on to
wilder lovemaking

DAY *364* THE RECKLESS GRASP

Forget everything but the drama of your bodies

a wild embrace for passionate reunions

*Relax into your beloved
in absolute safety*

make love, pleasure
her with your hands,
or just cuddle happily

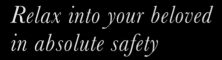

Random Selectors

In the mood for...
True Tenderness

7	321	17	76	276	179	112	14	225
174	127	333	90	2	291	123	311	322
338	52	97	82	184	55	305	86	244
137	211	345	170	217	138	347	70	286
1	257	36	234	94	226	24	281	18
328	104	358	68	155	249	339	95	128
144	77	309	131	246	125	43	77	297
45	185	19	224	4	320	194	255	175

In the mood for...
Deep Abandon

205	61	40	129	250	10	117	139	245
13	272	181	337	25	229	124	80	19
302	84	232	108	359	91	253	224	360
178	221	3	275	156	218	21	238	148
351	119	67	203	50	260	187	106	92
22	243	312	62	359	113	273	248	64
258	8	122	292	180	126	60	173	310
37	247	199	172	6	146	210	9	158

In the mood for...
Playful Moments

47	207	115	317	28	246	150	286	10
340	9	270	57	241	191	85	46	336
11	226	141	357	195	15	266	81	159
251	177	35	171	99	349	78	143	296
198	88	299	5	324	206	8	223	116
307	161	20	334	182	128	363	73	308
29	58	287	132	44	353	107	269	23
190	7	200	75	216	17	293	142	242

In the mood for...
Advanced Ecstasies

33	289	209	26	325	193	63	224	215
154	135	71	354	167	51	262	134	100
259	87	348	145	83	295	120	16	271
15	323	121	5	361	212	342	318	196
352	3	192	316	188	102	223	126	350
103	96	335	133	4	326	53	303	157
228	291	169	69	310	183	265	74	230
59	220	27	152	117	13	140	256	39

In the mood for...
Peaceful Embraces

9	300	236	76	283	42	314	277	70
329	14	340	213	163	194	12	184	234
231	362	305	6	265	254	105	227	299
355	166	93	240	311	56	191	365	18
32	286	318	281	101	226	114	89	345
346	2	202	130	233	82	247	294	237
162	328	276	48	269	257	66	333	309
267	54	111	282	1	147	288	31	214

In the mood for...
Uncommon Pleasures

109	261	239	65	284	176	332	30	252
285	12	327	279	204	293	201	264	165
160	343	189	136	341	41	348	149	92
301	79	298	81	186	304	222	319	219
235	331	49	268	316	98	344	118	313
356	151	315	197	164	330	72	278	230
34	280	274	364	11	262	208	306	16
263	229	168	38	260	110	290	153	184

ACKNOWLEDGMENTS

DK would like to thank John Rowley (photographer), Russell Burton and Gianni Mosella (assistants to photographer), Rhiannon Llewelyn and Kat Mead (photography direction), Peter Mallory (photography production) and Enzo Volpe (hair and makeup).

Special thanks to Kesta Desmond.